PRAISE FOR
the colorful kitchen

"Ilene has us covered with every color in the rainbow! These recipes are loaded with nutrition that haven't sacrificed any of the yummy flavor. From Coconut-Crusted Avocado Fries and Whole Roasted Tahini Cauliflower to Cheesy Broccoli & Bacon Stuffed Potatoes and Classic Chocolate Chip Cookies, every recipe is easy and delicious."
—Chloe Coscarelli, vegan chef and cookbook author of *Chloe Flavor*

"*The Colorful Kitchen* proves that plant-based cooking can be delicious, easy, and totally affordable. Ilene's beautiful recipes will leave you inspired, no matter how veggie-skeptical you are. A true feast for your belly and eyes!"
—Jessica Murnane, author of *One Part Plant* and host of the *One Part Podcast*

"If you've ever felt like eating more plants is blah or takes way too much time and effort until 'ta-da,' then Ilene's book is about to blow the tops off your carrots! With drool-worthy vegan dishes that truly taste as good as they look (trust me, I've been a long-time taste tester), *The Colorful Kitchen* should be a staple on your bookshelf that'll easily make plants a staple in your diet."
—Talia Pollock, founder of Party in My Plants and host of the *Party in My Plants Podcast*

the Colorful kitchen

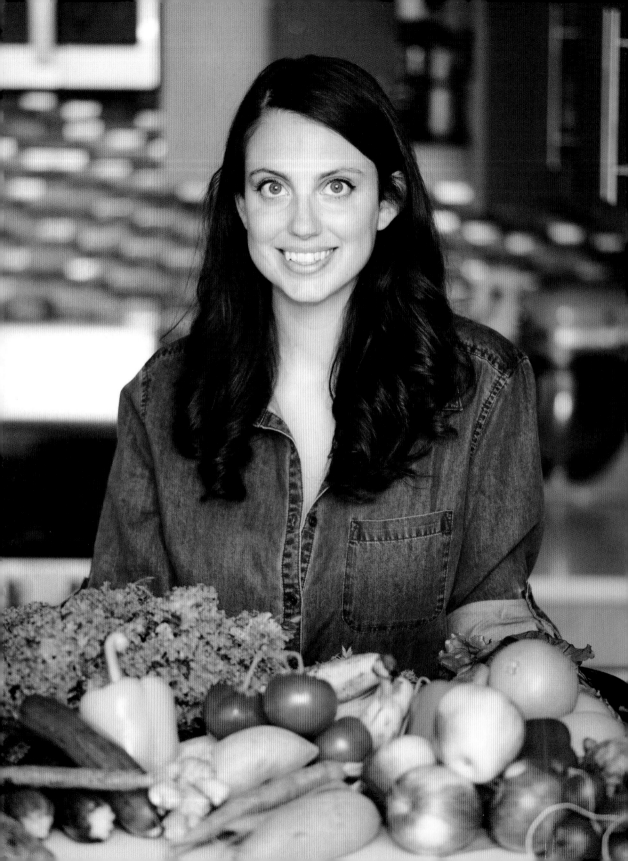

the Colorful kitchen

SIMPLE PLANT-BASED RECIPES FOR VIBRANCY, INSIDE AND OUT

ILENE GODOFSKY MORENO

BENBELLA BOOKS, INC.
DALLAS, TX

BenBella Books, Inc.
10440 N. Central Expressway, Suite 800
Dallas, TX 75231
www.benbellabooks.com
Send feedback to feedback@benbellabooks.com

Printed in the United States of America
10 9 8 7 6 5 4 3 2 1

Library of Congress Cataloging-in-Publication Data
Names: Moreno, Ilene Godofsky, author.
Title: The colorful kitchen : simple plant-based recipes for vibrancy, inside
   and out / Ilene Godofsky Moreno.
Description: Dallas, TX : BenBella Books, Inc., [2017] | Includes
   bibliographical references and index.
Identifiers: LCCN 2017019668 (print) | LCCN 2017037622 (ebook) | ISBN
   9781944648428 (electronic) | ISBN 9781944648411 (trade paper : alk. paper)
Subjects: LCSH: Cooking (Natural foods) | Nutrition. | Vegan cooking. |
   LCGFT: Cookbooks.
Classification: LCC TX741 (ebook) | LCC TX741 .A27 2017 (print) | DDC
   641.5/63—dc23
LC record available at https://lccn.loc.gov/2017019668

Editing by Maria Hart
Copyediting by Jennifer Brett Greenstein
Proofreading by Karen Wise and
   Rachel Phares
Indexing by WordCo Indexing Services, Inc.

Lifestyle photography by Alexa Drew Photography
Food photography by Ilene Godofsky Moreno
Cover design by Sarah Avinger
Text design and composition by Kit Sweeney
Printed by Versa Press

Distributed by Two Rivers Distribution
www.TwoRiversDistribution.com

To place orders through Two Rivers Distribution:
Tel: (800) 343-4499
Fax: (800) 351-5073
Email: pd_orderentry@ingramcontent.com

*Special discounts for bulk sales (minimum of 25 copies) are available.
Please contact Aida Herrera at aida@benbellabooks.com.*

For Violet and Ross,

MY FAVORITE PEOPLE TO EAT DINNER WITH

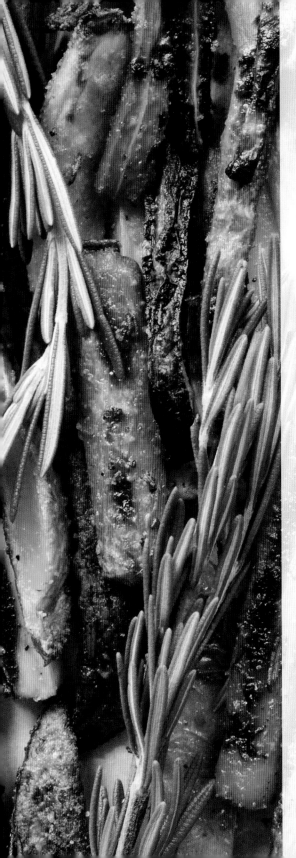

contents

my story

If you spend a few minutes looking at my blog, you might imagine that I was born into the kind of family who picked organic kale from their garden every morning, blended up green smoothies before they were hip, and spent Sunday afternoons baking granola together. But the truth is my beginnings couldn't be farther from this picture of a family enjoying healthy, natural foods; in fact, I spent the first two decades of my life eating anything but.

I grew up in a family that loved to eat, with parents who did *not* love to cook. That meant we ate the way many Americans did in the '80s, '90s, and early 2000s. We had takeout or made meals at home from processed ingredients that were designed to make cooking faster and easier, often by cutting out nutrients and pumping up the chemical preservatives.

A typical day of eating for us started with Pop-Tarts on the way out the door for breakfast, Happy Meals from the McDonald's drive-through for lunch, hot dogs and baked beans for dinner, and SnackWell's ("healthy") cookies for dessert.

There was always a half-eaten box of Cheez-It crackers or Entenmann's cookies open on the counter that we grazed on throughout the day. Our diet was far from the picture of health. But my family did get one thing spot-on: my mom, dad, younger brother, and I always sat down at the table to eat dinner together—and that provided another kind of very important nourishment.

When I was nine years old, I saw a live lobster cooked in a pot of boiling water and a lightbulb went off in my head: *The food on my plate used to be a real, living animal!* I immediately declared myself a vegetarian.

My parents were initially skeptical, but after much foot stomping on my end, they eventually became supportive. Still, they had no idea what to feed me. I wasn't interested in vegetables, which meant I usually ended up eating grilled cheese sandwiches and the occasional frozen veggie burger. My diet quickly shrank to cheese, bread, and mashed potatoes. At the insistence of my mother, I included iceberg lettuce, which I'd drown in an entire bottle of ranch dressing in the name of "salad."

My stint as a vegetarian didn't last very long, and for almost ten years I would fall into the pattern of avoiding meat for a few weeks before quickly tiring of my options and resuming my family's Standard American Diet. Eating chicken nuggets and Hamburger Helper with my family was so much easier than finding meat-free foods that I actually liked. It wasn't until my freshman year of art school that my vegetarianism finally stuck. With just a microwave and a mini-fridge in my dorm room, and 24/7 access to French fries and frozen yogurt at the school cafeteria, I had become a full-fledged, veggie-burger-nuking, grilled-cheese-every-night, junk-food-loving vegetarian.

I ate tons of dairy, processed food, and frozen faux-meat products. I found the taste of most fruit to be too intense; it lacked the watered-down and artificial flavors of the "fruit"-flavored gummy bears and candy that I was used to, and the natural combination of sweet and tart was too much for me. Green vegetables were out of the question unless they were smothered in cheese. One night I decided that I was going to cook "something healthy" for dinner, so I put a whole head of broccoli in the microwave, topped it with cheese slices, and nuked it for three minutes. Yep, it was *that* bad.

At the same time that I was dousing anything green in vats of cheese, I used to have a lot of allergies. For as long as I could remember, sneezing, wheezing, and congestion were a part of my daily life. I was always on multiple prescription medications that seemed to do little more than make me drowsy. On top of that, I had an assortment of digestive issues, and I thought it was normal to have a stomachache after each meal. Overall, I felt generally "not great" every day.

At age twenty, I was studying textile design at the Rhode Island School of Design. RISD is known for its heavy workload and six-hour critiques that frequently end in tears. Between all-night work sessions and covering myself in head-to-toe glitter for weekend parties (art school students know how to party!), I began to wonder if it was possible to feel better than "not great" every day.

Years before, I had heard about a friend of a friend with an aunt who supposedly cured herself of cancer by going on a macrobiotic diet. After her miraculous recovery, her whole family adopted the diet and all their ailments disappeared as well. I was pretty sure the story was a major exaggeration, and macrobiotics sounded like an extreme health-nut diet to me, but by this point my energy was sputtering and I was desperate, so I decided to give it a try.

A macrobiotic diet typically includes lots of whole grains, cooked vegetables, and legumes—everything I didn't eat—with little to no meat, dairy, sugar, or processed food—everything (except the meat) that I did. I picked a few recipes from a cookbook, went to the health-food store, and bought a basket full of ingredients that were totally new to me. It was 2007, when green juice, kale chips, and quinoa were still a few years away from becoming trendy, so I felt like I was grocery shopping on a different planet.

The first few days of cooking and eating this way were eye-opening. Shockingly, I actually liked the taste of the food I was eating. By the fourth day of munching on veggies, beans, and grains, I started to feel a sense of lightness and clarity that I had never felt before. By the end of the first month, my stomachaches and allergies had completely disappeared and I was able to go off all my medications. It honestly felt like magic: I had energy, my skin was clear, I had shed a little extra weight, and I felt like a newly minted human being.

The downside was that I was spending hours and hours following complicated recipes when I should have been working on my studies, and blowing way too much money on fancy ingredients. When it felt like too much effort to make dinner, I would resort to a plate of brown rice, plain tofu, and steamed broccoli—exactly the kind of tasteless, boring meal that gives vegan food a bad reputation. My friends and family definitely thought I had become a full-fledged health weirdo, and I found myself skipping out on social events where I was afraid there wouldn't be anything for me to eat. As for dating, my thoughts on the subject were, *Sure, I would love to go on a date with you! As long as you don't mind if I bring my own dinner to the restaurant and we spend two hours talking about the benefits of presoaking grains.* In short, I

was completely consumed by the food I was consuming.

The summer rolled around and I found myself working as an intern at a fabric-design company in Manhattan. My schedule was much less rigorous than it had been at school, and I suddenly had the free time and mental space to take a step back and look at how my diet was affecting my life. On one hand, I absolutely loved the way I felt (no more daily stomachaches or sniffles), but I also had a feeling that it shouldn't take so much of my time, money, and social life to feel this way.

I decided to experiment with ingredients outside the typical macrobiotic diet and started adding in other plant-based foods (fruit, raw vegetables, nuts, and so on). Suddenly I was having more fun coming up with creative meals and relying less on the recipes in my cookbooks. After some trial and error (and many really unfortunate dishes), I realized that I didn't need fancy kitchen equipment or exotic ingredients to put together a great meal. I ate what I liked and I finally liked *real* food. I learned to listen to my body and continued experimenting with which foods helped me feel my best (spoiler alert: plants and unprocessed food did the trick), and I taught myself to make recipes that were *colorful, not complicated,* which became my mantra.

Along the way I continued to learn about the issues of animal cruelty and environmental sustainability facing the meat, dairy, and egg industries. Nourishing my body with a plant-based diet felt even better when I knew that I was also being kind to the planet and all its inhabitants.

At first it was difficult for many of my friends and family to understand why I ate the way I did. As I became more and more comfortable in the kitchen, it became easier for me to explain why I was happy no longer covering everything in cheese and skipping turkey at Thanksgiving. I'd simply make one of my favorite dishes and let the food speak for itself. Eating became social for me again. I loved hosting dinner parties and bringing my creations to potlucks. I found that I could order something plant-based at almost every restaurant, so I never had to skip a friend's birthday dinner again. I even started dating my now-husband Ross, and didn't scare him away by constantly chatting about leafy greens.

In 2013, five years after I picked up my first macrobiotic cookbook, I started my blog *The Colorful Kitchen*. Thanks to my education in art and my career in the textile industry, I began to approach cooking the same way I approached my design work. I viewed each meal through a designer's lens and started utilizing elements like texture, balance, and color to create recipes that were both visually inviting and delicious. I started to think of my plate as a blank canvas, and I wanted to fill it with food that was exciting at first sight, with flavors and textures that came together harmoniously. Above all else, I wanted people to look at the photos on my blog, say "That looks delicious!" and then actually make the recipes because the instructions are so doable.

It's now been ten years since I started my journey toward a healthier lifestyle and a diet filled with vibrant color. By listening to my body, enjoying seasonal produce, and eating the food I actually like, I never get bored. Each meal is still an exciting opportunity to fill my plate with color.

Enjoying food that makes me feel my best is no longer a reclusive activity. Being able to share vibrant meals with my friends, family, and readers provides nourishment that goes deeper than just the food on my plate.

COLORFUL, NOT COMPLICATED

Why the emphasis on *colorful* food? Different-colored fruits and vegetables contain different vitamins and minerals, but beyond that, food that looks great simply tastes better. Have you ever finished a big meal but still felt hungry afterward? I can think of so many times when I made a delicious (but monochromatic and visually boring) recipe, like a bowl of lentil soup, and found myself poking around the fridge afterward. The meal was hearty and tasted great, but I was left unsatisfied because my eyes didn't get a chance to eat. These days, I'll make the same soup, but top it with a dollop of **Cashew Sour Cream** (see page 226), a forkful of red sauerkraut, and a sprinkle of parsley and—voila!—I have a gorgeous bowl to dig in to, and I feel completely satiated afterward.

When you fill your plate with a rainbow of colors, you're not only adding flavor, texture, and visual appeal but also filling your plate with nutrients. Counting colors is way more fun than counting calories, carbs, and fat. Beginning a meal by saying "This looks delicious!" rather than "I wonder how many calories are in this?" helps cultivate a healthier relationship with food. When you eat whole foods and your meals taste *and* look delicious (and you know everything on your plate is great for you without having to crunch any numbers), the experience of cooking and eating is even more nourishing.

MY KITCHEN

Back when I first started my blog, my friends were always surprised that the recipes I posted were actually coming out of my shabby kitchen. My kitchen was about half the size of my current one and not the least bit fancy. The floors were far from level and the door to the only bathroom in the apartment was right next to the refrigerator. There was no pantry, so I crowded the walls with shelves, where I stored all the bulk foods in mason jars. Even without an inch of counter space to spare or a dishwasher to help with cleanup, I managed to put together every single recipe in this book.

I was fortunate to receive many of my dream kitchen gadgets (pricey blender, stand mixer, and so on) as wedding gifts, but for the first few years of *The Colorful Kitchen* blog, I got by with a mismatched, bare-bones assortment of hand-me-down equipment and dishes.

As much fun as froufrou kitchen gadgets can be, you won't need any of them for the recipes in this book. In fact, you probably already have everything you need. As long as you've got a blender, a couple of different-sized pots and pans, a good knife, and a few spatulas and mixing spoons, you're good to go. A food processor and electric mixer are also great if you have them, but you can easily make do by chopping and mixing by hand.

SAVE TIME BY COOKING MULTIPLE MEALS AT ONCE

One of the easiest ways to enjoy homemade food *and* cut down on how much time you're spending in the kitchen

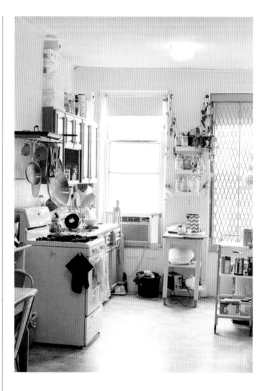

is to cook more than one meal at a time. One way to do this is to simply double what you're making for dinner and enjoy it for lunch the next day. When I'm especially busy, I like to make a few dishes on Sunday night, so all I have to do is heat them up throughout the week. I'm also a big fan of doubling, tripling, or even quadrupling recipes, then freezing individual portions for nights when I'm short on time.

That said, my favorite way to save time and still enjoy a variety of different recipes is to find multiple ways to use one element. You'll notice that many of the recipes in this book share sauces, dressings, or other components. For example, the **Green Cashew Ranch Dressing** (see page 234) that's drizzled over the **Southwestern Salad** (see page 77) is also used as the dipping sauce for the **BBQ Cauliflower**

Poppers (see page 135), and it replaces the traditional mayo in the **Loaded Ranch Potato Salad** (see page 136). By planning ahead, you can triple the amount of dressing you make and easily whip up three different recipes using the same sauce over the course of a week.

Look for the ⊕ symbol, which indicates a recipe uses another recipe in the book.

If you don't usually plan your weekly menu in advance, thinking about cooking this way can certainly feel overwhelming at first. Start by just trying out one week of batch cooking, and you'll notice that you're spending less time wondering what to make for dinner, less time cooking, and more time enjoying colorful meals.

MAKE MY RECIPES YOUR OWN

My hope for you, dear reader, is that the recipes in this book will provide a starting point for you to express your own creativity through cooking. Whether you're cooking for one, two, or twelve, these recipes are designed to give you a foundation from which to embark on your own colorful journey in the kitchen.

These are the recipes I wish I had in my toolbox all those years ago when preparing a healthy dinner felt like too much work. Use them as a template and add whatever ingredients are in season and fresh. Don't be afraid to make substitutions and additions—and when in doubt, always add avocado.

colorful ingredient guide

You'll probably find most of the ingredients in this book easy, familiar, and available wherever you shop for groceries. Below are explanations of why I opt for certain ingredients as well as descriptions of a few you may not be familiar with.

BREAD For toast and sandwiches, I like to use a spelt loaf from my local bakery. Many people find spelt to be easier on their stomachs than wheat. For gluten-free options, check your own local bakeries or health-food stores (the freezer section is always a good bet).

CACAO A few recipes call for cacao powder and cacao nibs. Cacao is chocolate in its raw form. It has a slightly different flavor and a higher antioxidant power than its processed counterpart, cocoa.

COCONUT BUTTER Also called coconut manna, coconut butter is a creamy spread made from pureed coconut meat, and it's a good creamy swap for dairy butter.

COCONUT SUGAR For baked goods, I prefer coconut sugar over refined white sugar because it has a lower glycemic index and contains small amounts of vitamins and minerals—plus I love its rich, caramel-like flavor.

FLAXSEED Flaxseed packs a high nutritional punch and provides tons of fiber, which is why I love to add it to breakfast recipes like smoothies and oatmeal. It also acts as a binding agent, which is why you'll find a flax "egg" used in many recipes (especially baked goods).

FROZEN BANANAS I always keep bananas in my freezer so I can whip up a smoothie or quick ice cream (see pages 19 and 218) at any time. The best way to freeze bananas is to peel and slice them into 1-inch pieces, place the pieces on a baking sheet lined with parchment paper, and throw them in the freezer. Allow the bananas to freeze on the baking sheet for 2 hours, and then transfer them to an airtight container and store in the freezer until needed.

FULL-FAT CANNED COCONUT MILK Pay special attention to recipes that call for full-fat canned coconut milk and don't skimp! Reduced-fat versions are not as thick and creamy and could cause your recipes to flop.

LEMON JUICE I always keep lemons on hand because fresh lemon juice is one of the easiest ways to add flavor to almost any dish. Many of the recipes in this book call for the juice of one whole lemon, which is about 3 tablespoons. Fresh lemon juice is best, but if you're feeling a little lazy you can buy a bottle of pure lemon juice and quickly measure it out.

LIQUID SMOKE This is my secret ingredient for making the most delicious veggie burgers and tempeh "bacon." Just a couple of drops add an open-flame flavor to any dish.

MAPLE SYRUP Maple syrup is my favorite liquid sweetener. It's used in many of the dessert recipes, as well as the sauces and dressings, for a touch of sweetness. Agave, brown rice syrup, or date syrup can also be an easy swap, but you may need a slightly smaller or larger amount.

NONDAIRY MILK Almond milk, especially homemade (see page 223), is my personal favorite because of its creaminess. But soy, oat, rice, and coconut milk are also great options, and all are increasingly found at regular grocery stores if you don't want to make your own.

NUTRITIONAL YEAST Nutritional yeast is a dairy-free secret weapon that easily adds a cheesy flavor to any dish, plus it's full of vitamin B12. I like to use it in sauces or sprinkle it on top of salads and pasta as a Parmesan cheese substitute.

PASTA I usually use gluten-free brown rice pasta because I love the texture, but feel free to use whatever kind you prefer.

PEANUT BUTTER For simplicity's sake (and for the sake of my wallet), peanut is my nut butter of choice for the recipes in this book. Feel free to swap it out for almond, cashew, or any other nut butter.

ROLLED OATS My oatmeal recipes and some of the baked goods call for rolled oats. I opt for rolled oats because they cook faster than steel-cut oats and have a better texture than instant oats.

SOAKED CASHEWS Wondering why so many recipes call for cashews soaked in water? Not only does soaking nuts help them become easier to digest, but it also softens them, making for super-creamy blended sauces, soups, and desserts. A few of the recipes call for cashews soaked for at least 4 hours. You can speed this up by soaking them in hot water and/or using a high-speed blender.

SPELT FLOUR As a cousin of wheat, spelt is not gluten-free, but it does contain a lower amount of gluten. Many people, like me, find it easier to digest than wheat.

TAMARI Tamari is gluten-free soy sauce. Feel free to substitute regular soy sauce, Bragg Liquid Aminos, or coconut aminos in any recipes that call for tamari.

TEMPEH I like to think of tempeh as tofu's heartier cousin. Made from fermented soybeans, tempeh has a nutty flavor and meaty texture and adds easy protein to any meal.

TOFU Even though it's become much more mainstream in recent years, I know many people who are scared of cooking with tofu. My **Baked Tofu** (see page 233) is a great place for tofu newbies to start.

VEGAN CHEESE, VEGAN MAYO, AND VEGAN BUTTER It's truly incredible how many vegan substitutes have hit the dairy section in the past few years. While most of the recipes in this book don't depend on processed foods like these as main ingredients, they can be a quick and easy way to add flavor.

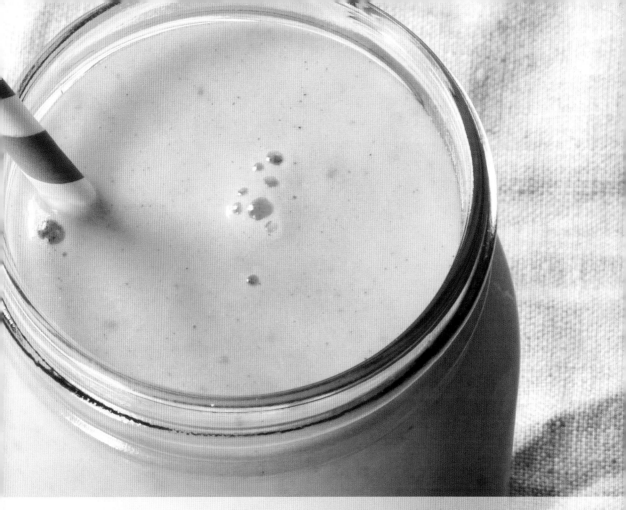

smoothies

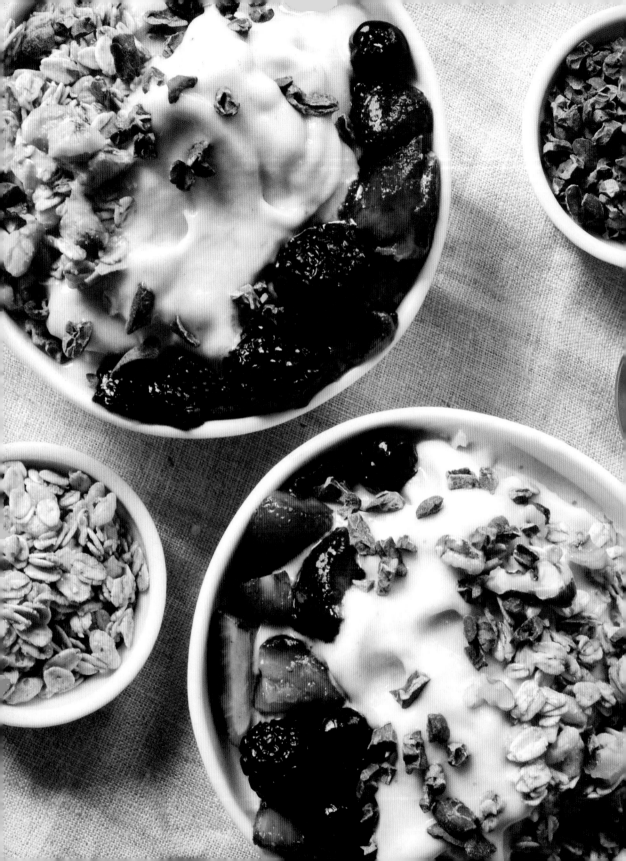

BANANA BREAKFAST
ice cream SUNDAE

⊕ **TOTAL TIME:** 5 MINUTES **MAKES:** 2 SERVINGS

Just like a DIY frozen yogurt bar (but for breakfast!), this is a really fun recipe because you can pile on all the toppings you love and skip the ones you don't (I'm looking at you, gummy worms).

ICE CREAM
2–3 frozen bananas*
Nondairy milk, as needed
　to blend

TOPPINGS
½ cup mixed berries
½ cup granola, store-bought
　or homemade (see
　pages 49–52)
2 tablespoons cacao nibs
Any other nuts, seeds, or
　superfoods you like

1. To prepare the ice cream, combine the bananas and 1 tablespoon of nondairy milk in a blender or food processor. Blend, adding 1 tablespoon of milk at a time, as needed, until a texture similar to that of frozen yogurt is formed.

2. Transfer the ice cream to bowls, add the toppings, and enjoy right away.

NOTE: *See how to freeze bananas in the* **Colorful Ingredient Guide** *(page 16).*

pink & purple
COCONUT SMOOTHIE

TOTAL TIME: 5 MINUTES **MAKES:** 2 SERVINGS

I love gawking at photos of smoothies on Instagram that are made of seven different-colored layers, spilling out of their mason jars with a perfect pile of superfoods and edible flowers on top. The few times I've tried my hand at making one of these creations, I quickly realized it would take me forty-five minutes to pull it together—which is way too long to wait for breakfast—and it simply was not worth the effort. With two layers, this delicious and pretty smoothie will only take a few minutes of your time, but it will still totally impress on Instagram, so get out your phone!

2 cups coconut water
2 frozen bananas*
1 cup frozen raspberries and/or strawberries
2 tablespoons coconut butter
1 cup frozen blueberries and/or blackberries

1. To prepare the pink layer, combine the coconut water, bananas, raspberries and/or strawberries, and coconut butter in a blender and blend until smooth.

2. Transfer two-thirds of the smoothie to glasses.

3. To prepare the purple layer, add the blueberries and/or blackberries to the blender and blend until smooth.

4. Pour the purple layer on top of the pink layer in the glasses and enjoy.

NOTE: *See how to freeze bananas in the* **Colorful Ingredient Guide** *(page 16).*

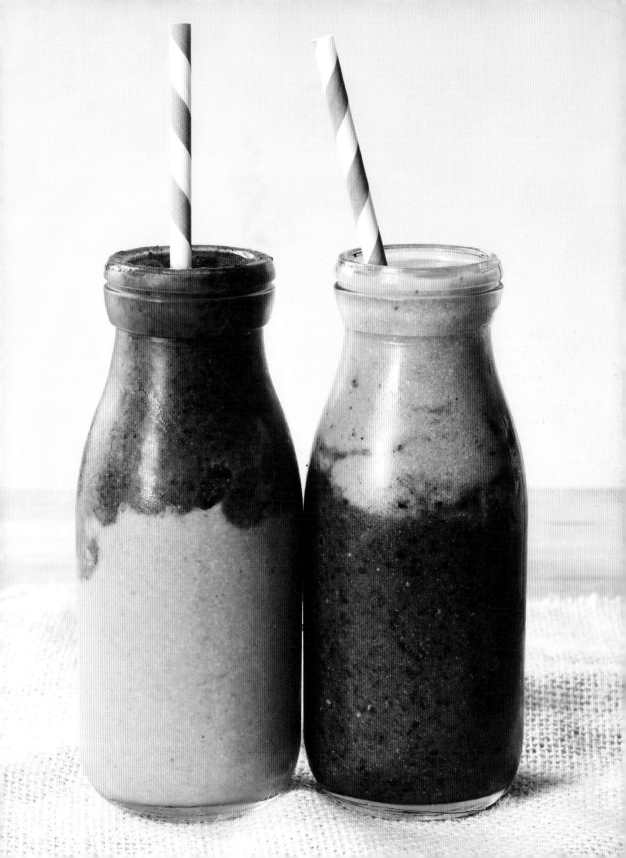

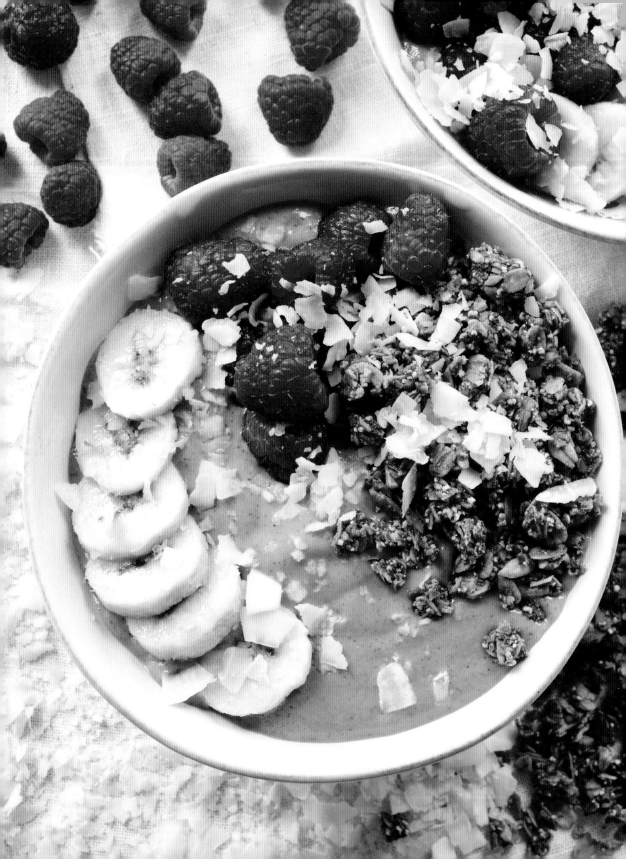

GO-TO *green smoothie*

TOTAL TIME: 5 MINUTES **MAKES:** 2 SERVINGS

For years, I've been sharing this recipe with friends and blog readers who ask me for a smoothie recipe that will actually keep them full until lunch. It's also a great template for smoothie newbies: start here and swap in different kinds of nut butters, greens, and frozen fruits.

2 bananas (use frozen bananas* for a colder, thicker smoothie)

1 cup frozen fruit (pineapple, mango, berries, etc.)

2 tablespoons ground flaxseed

2 tablespoons peanut butter

1 cup packed kale

1½ cups nondairy milk

1. Combine all the ingredients in a blender and blend until smooth.

2. Transfer to glasses to serve.

NOTE: *See how to freeze bananas in the* **Colorful Ingredient Guide** *(page 16).*

MAKE IT A . . . GO-TO GREEN SMOOTHIE BOWL

TOTAL TIME: 5 MINUTES
MAKES: 2 SERVINGS

For some of us, even the most filling smoothies don't feel like a full meal. To make it extra hearty, make it a bowl!

1 batch Go-To Green Smoothie

1 banana, sliced

1 cup fresh berries

½ cup granola, store-bought or homemade (see pages 49–52)

2 tablespoons shredded coconut

1. Transfer the **Go-To Green Smoothie** to bowls.

2. Top with the banana, berries, granola, and coconut and enjoy with a spoon.

CHOCOLATE *superfood* SMOOTHIE

⊕ **TOTAL TIME:** 5 MINUTES **MAKES:** 2 SERVINGS

This smoothie is for the times when your sweet tooth says "milkshake" but your brain says "salad"! It tastes decadent enough for dessert, but it's secretly wholesome enough for breakfast.

SMOOTHIE
1 frozen banana*
1 avocado, pitted and scooped
1½ cups nondairy milk
1 cup packed spinach
3 Medjool dates, pitted*
¼ cup cacao or cocoa powder
2 tablespoons maple syrup
2 tablespoons chia seeds

TOPPINGS
¼ batch Coconut Whipped
   Cream (see page 227) or
   Sweet Cashew Cream (see
   page 224)
2 tablespoons cacao nibs

1. Combine all the smoothie ingredients in a blender and blend until smooth.

2. Transfer to glasses. Add the **Coconut Whipped Cream** or **Sweet Cashew Cream** and cacao nibs on top.

NOTE: *See how to freeze bananas in the Colorful Ingredient Guide (page 16).*

NOTE: *If you aren't using a high-speed blender, you may want to soften the dates by soaking them in hot water for 5 minutes so they blend smoothly.*

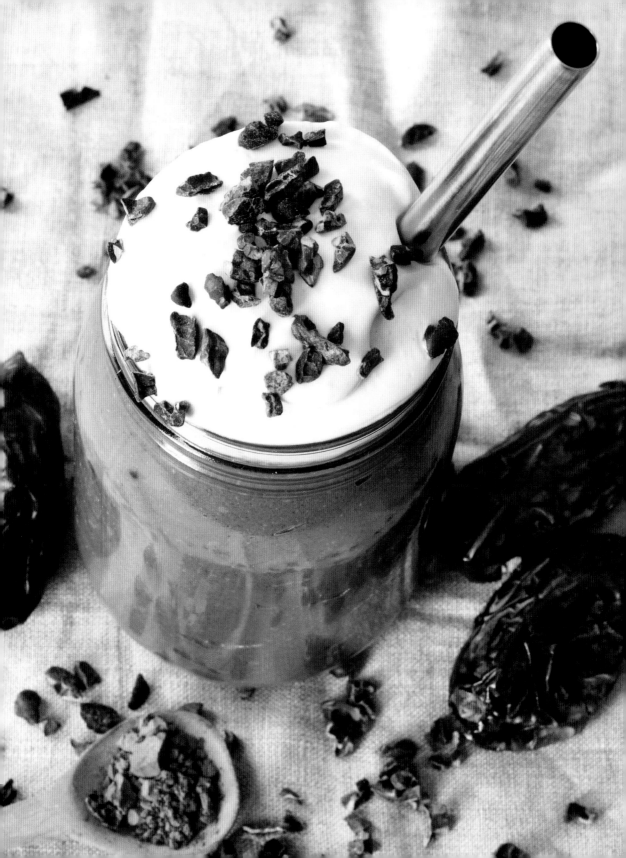

tropical SMOOTHIE PARFAIT

TOTAL TIME: 5 MINUTES **MAKES:** 2 SERVINGS

As a New Yorker, throughout the year I look forward to summer in the city. When it's snowing outside I daydream about biking along the water, outdoor concerts, and rooftop movie nights. But by the second week in June, the reality always sets in that summer in the city actually means stinky streets, subway rides without air-conditioning, and sweaty climbs to fifth-floor apartments. Staying cool becomes a full-time job and one of my favorite tricks is stationing myself in front a fan with this yummy smoothie in hand.

SMOOTHIE
2 cups frozen pineapple chunks
2 cups frozen mango chunks
1½ cups orange juice

EVERYTHING ELSE
⅔ cup granola, store-bought or homemade (see pages 49–52)
1 cup fresh fruit (berries, sliced bananas, etc.)
2 tablespoons shredded coconut

1. Combine the smoothie ingredients in a blender and blend until smooth.

2. Fill glasses halfway with the smoothie. Add a layer of granola, then fill the glasses with the remaining smoothie.

3. Top with the remaining granola and the fruit and coconut.

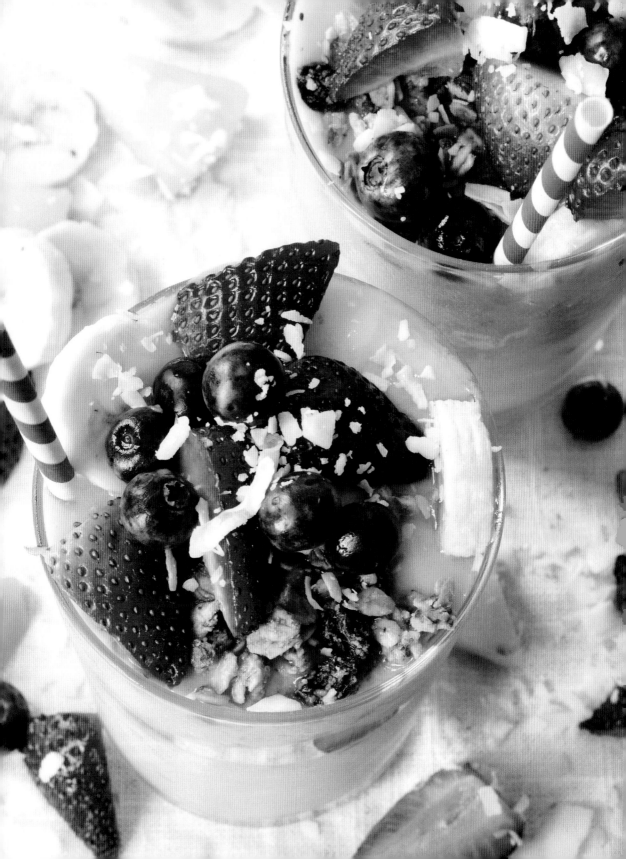

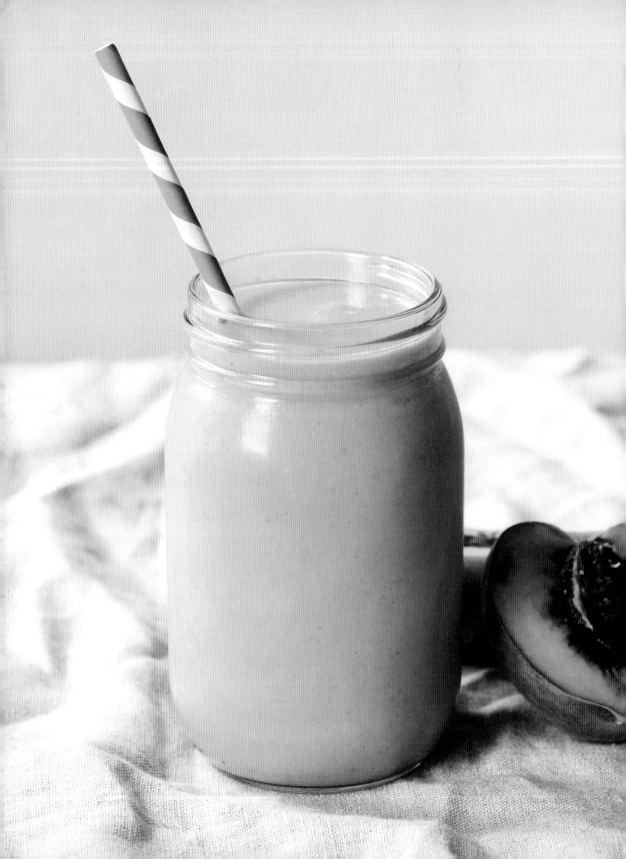

PEACHY TAHINI
sunshine SMOOTHIE

TOTAL TIME: 5 MINUTES   **MAKES:** 2 SERVINGS

I wish I could tell you how this recipe came to be, but my only explanation is that I first whipped it up while I was nine and a half months pregnant. The unanimous reaction to this recipe from my testers was that it sounded like a really weird list of ingredients, but they ended up being super-surprised by how much they liked it.

2 cups frozen peach slices
1½ cups nondairy milk
1 cup chopped carrots
2–3 medjool dates, pitted*
3 tablespoons tahini
¼ teaspoon ground cinnamon

1. Combine all the ingredients in a blender and blend until smooth.

2. Transfer to glasses to serve.

NOTE: *If you aren't using a high-speed blender, you may want to soften the dates by soaking them in hot water for 5 minutes so they blend smoothly.*

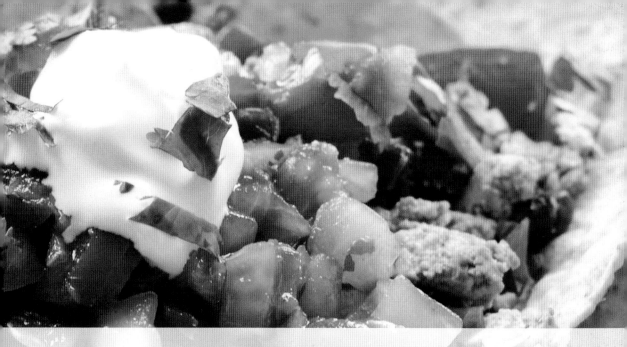

breakfast

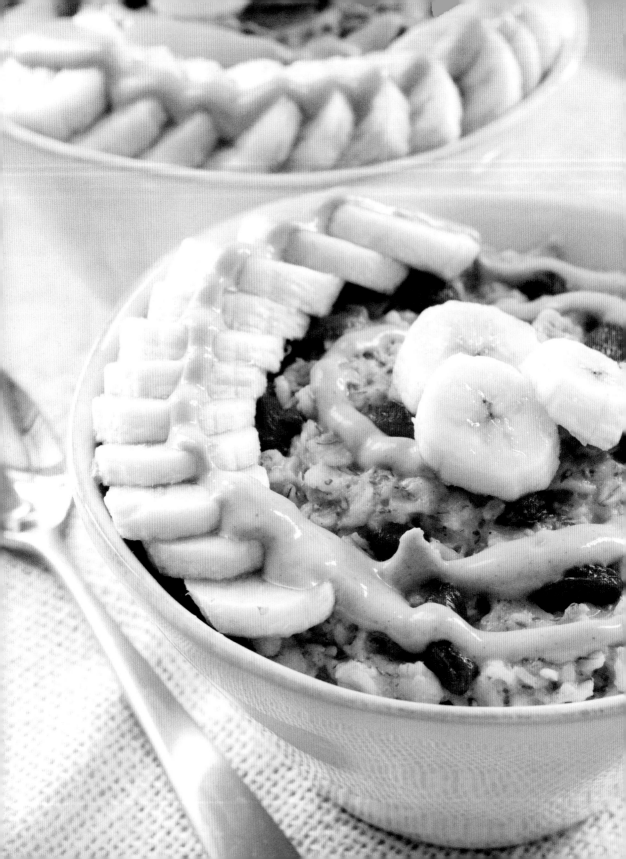

PEANUT BUTTER & BANANA *oatmeal*

TOTAL TIME: 10 MINUTES **MAKES:** 2 SERVINGS

I used to make oatmeal for my husband every morning for breakfast. Once I became pregnant with our daughter, I decided that it was his turn to make breakfast for me, so I taught him this super-easy recipe. If the man who has only cooked a handful of meals in his entire life can make this every morning, anyone can!

OATMEAL
1 cup rolled oats
1 cup nondairy milk
1 cup water
½ teaspoon vanilla extract
¼ cup raisins or goji berries
Dash of ground cinnamon
Dash of salt
2 tablespoons ground flaxseed

TOPPINGS
1 banana, sliced
2 tablespoons peanut butter

1. In a small pot over low heat, bring the oats, nondairy milk, and water to a simmer.

2. Stir in the vanilla extract, raisins or goji berries, cinnamon, and salt. Continue to simmer, stirring occasionally, until the liquid is absorbed, 7–10 minutes.

3. Turn off the heat and stir in the ground flaxseed. Transfer to bowls and add the toppings.

carrot cake OATMEAL

TOTAL TIME: 10 MINUTES **MAKES:** 2 SERVINGS

Do you wake up with a raging sweet tooth? Me too. Eating this filling oatmeal is like having carrot cake for breakfast, but it's full of ingredients that will get your day started off right.

OATMEAL
1 cup rolled oats
1 cup nondairy milk
1 cup water
½ cup shredded carrot
¼ cup raisins
½ teaspoon vanilla extract
½ teaspoon ground cinnamon
¼ teaspoon ground allspice
Dash of salt

TOPPINGS
2 tablespoons maple syrup
¼ cup chopped walnuts
2 tablespoons shredded
   coconut

1. In a small pot over low heat, bring the oats, nondairy milk, and water to a simmer.

2. Stir in the carrot, raisins, vanilla extract, cinnamon, allspice, and salt. Continue to simmer, stirring occasionally, until all the liquid is absorbed, 7–10 minutes.

3. Transfer to bowls, drizzle with maple syrup, and add the walnuts and coconut on top.

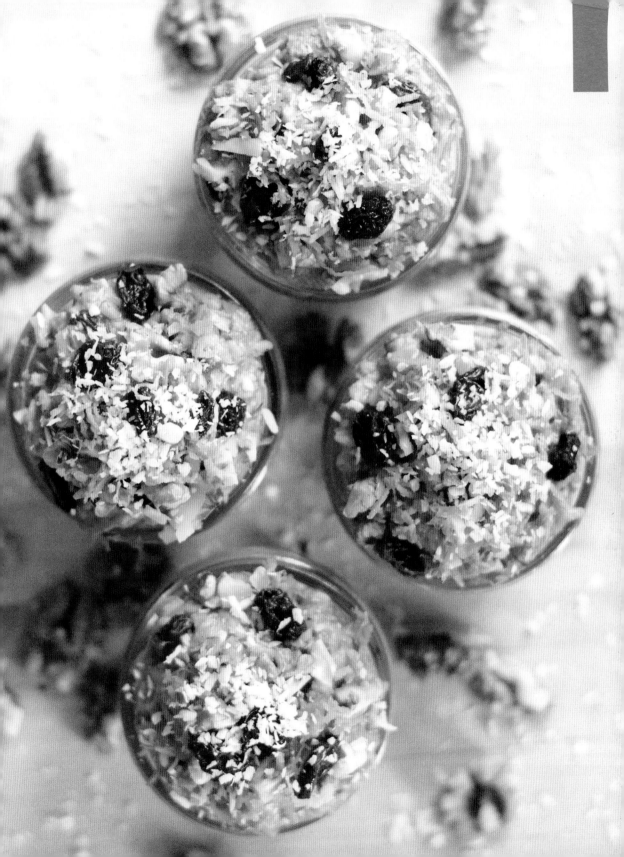

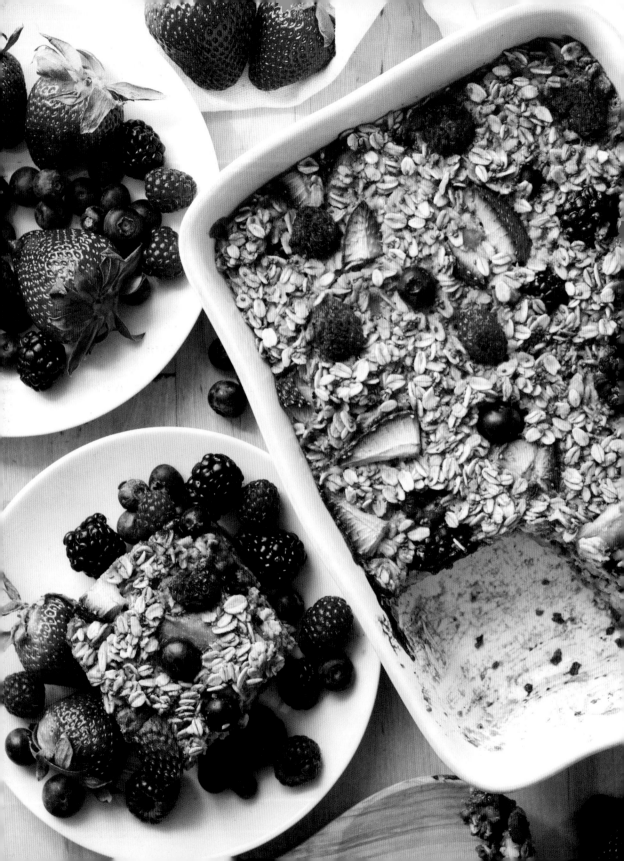

fruity BAKED OATMEAL

⊕ **TOTAL TIME:** 45 MINUTES **ACTIVE TIME:** 10 MINUTES **MAKES:** 6–8 SERVINGS

Say hello to your new brunch staple! I like to warm up weekend mornings with this oatmeal served right out of the oven. It's also great to slice, freeze, and heat up individual pieces for quick weekday breakfasts. Bonus points if you add a spoonful of peanut butter on top.

DRY
3 cups rolled oats
¼ cup chia seeds
1 teaspoon ground cinnamon
⅛ teaspoon salt

WET
3 cups nondairy milk
1 ripe medium banana, mashed
¼ cup maple syrup
1 tablespoon vanilla extract

FOLD-IN
1 cup mixed berries

TOPPING OPTIONS
1 batch Sweet Cashew Cream
   (see page 224)
1 batch Coconut Whipped
   Cream (see page 227)
Maple syrup to taste

1. Preheat the oven to 350°F. Grease a 10-by-7-inch or 8-by-8-inch glass baking dish.

2. In a large bowl, whisk the dry ingredients together. In a small bowl, stir the wet ingredients together. Add the contents of the small bowl to the large bowl and stir until thoroughly combined. Fold in the berries.

3. Transfer the mixture to the baking dish and use a spatula to spread it out evenly.

4. Bake for 35 minutes, or until the top is golden and crisp. Serve warm with the toppings.

JAZZY *avocado* TOAST

TOTAL TIME: 5 MINUTES **MAKES:** 2 SERVINGS

Who doesn't love avocado toast? I like this savory and slightly spicy version because it's filled with a range of textures thanks to creamy avocado, crispy toast, and crunchy pumpkin seeds.

2 slices of bread
1 avocado, sliced
Juice of ½ lemon
2 tablespoons pumpkin seeds
Dash of red pepper flakes
Dash of smoked paprika
Dash of sesame seeds
Dash of salt
Dash of black pepper

1. Toast the bread.

2. Layer the avocado slices on the toast.

3. Drizzle the lemon juice over the avocado. Sprinkle the pumpkin seeds, red pepper flakes, paprika, sesame seeds, salt, and black pepper on top, to taste.

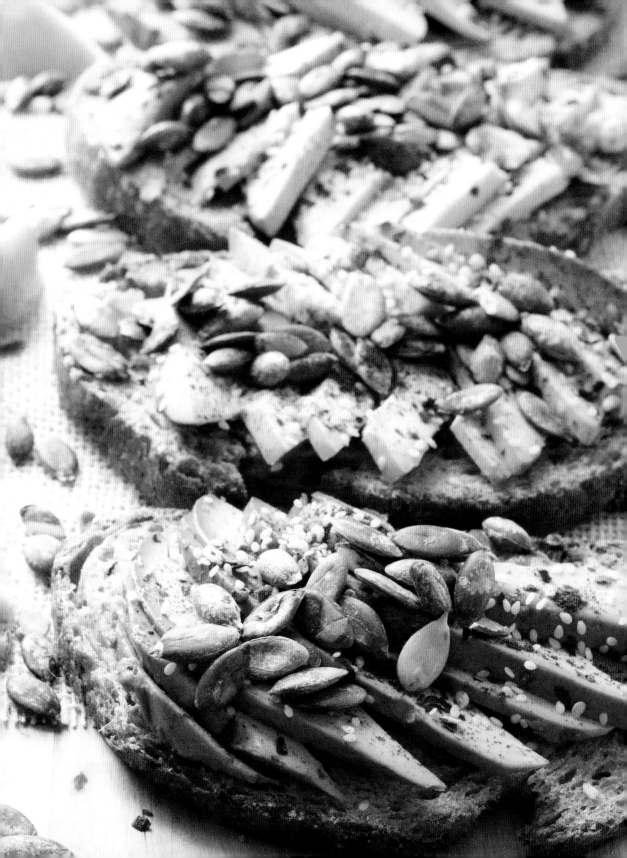

PB&J *sweet cream* TOAST

⊕ **TOTAL TIME:** 5 MINUTES **MAKES:** 2 SERVINGS

This toast is for kids of all ages who love PB&Js. With Sweet Cashew Cream, it's reminiscent of a Marshmallow Fluff sandwich—but without the sugar coma.

2 slices of bread
¼ batch Sweet Cashew Cream (see page 224)*
2 tablespoons jam or fruit preserves
2 tablespoons peanut butter

1. Toast the bread.

2. Layer the Sweet Cashew Cream, jam or preserves, and peanut butter on the toast.

NOTE: *Not sure what to do with the rest of your Sweet Cashew Cream? I like to add a dollop on top of my smoothies or dunk cookies into it.*

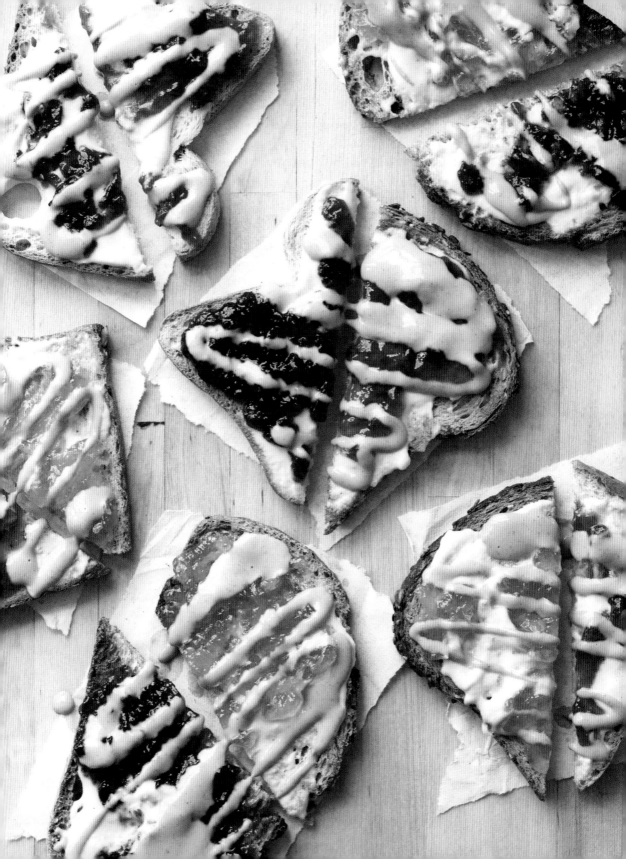

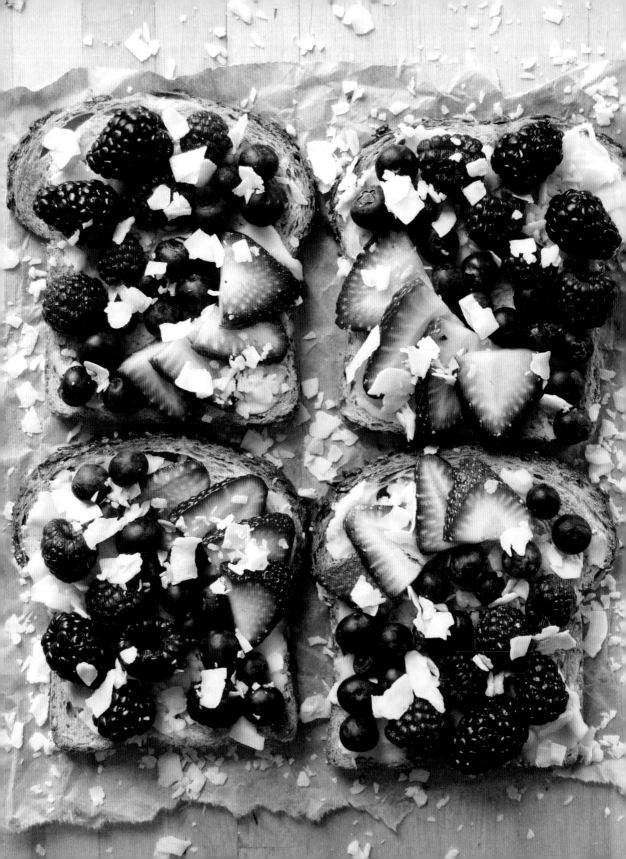

coconut BERRY TOAST

TOTAL TIME: 5 MINUTES **MAKES:** 2 SERVINGS

I've always loved all things coconut, but I only discovered coconut butter fairly recently. The way it melts on warm toast is a coconut lover's dream. One of my recipe testers described this dish as a cousin to French toast (thanks for making me feel fancy!). But it's much easier to make.

2 slices of bread
2 tablespoons coconut butter
½ cup mixed berries
2 tablespoons maple syrup
1 tablespoon shredded
    coconut
Dash of salt

1. Toast the bread.

2. Spread the coconut butter on the toast.

3. Layer the berries over the coconut butter. Drizzle the maple syrup on top, and sprinkle with the coconut and salt.

SAVORY
sweet potato TOAST

TOTAL TIME: 5 MINUTES   MAKES: 2 SERVINGS

Save your leftover sweet potato from dinner (see Sweet Potato Skins on page 173) and make this easy, satisfying toast the next morning for breakfast.

2 slices of bread
1 tablespoon olive oil
1 handful baby spinach
1 cup mashed cooked sweet potato (both warm and cold are delicious)
2 tablespoons sunflower seeds
2 tablespoons tahini
1 tablespoon chopped fresh parsley
Salt and black pepper, to taste

1. Toast the bread.

2. Drizzle the olive oil on the toast. Spread the spinach on top, then add the sweet potato.

3. Sprinkle the sunflower seeds and drizzle the tahini on top. Finish by topping with the parsley, salt, and pepper.

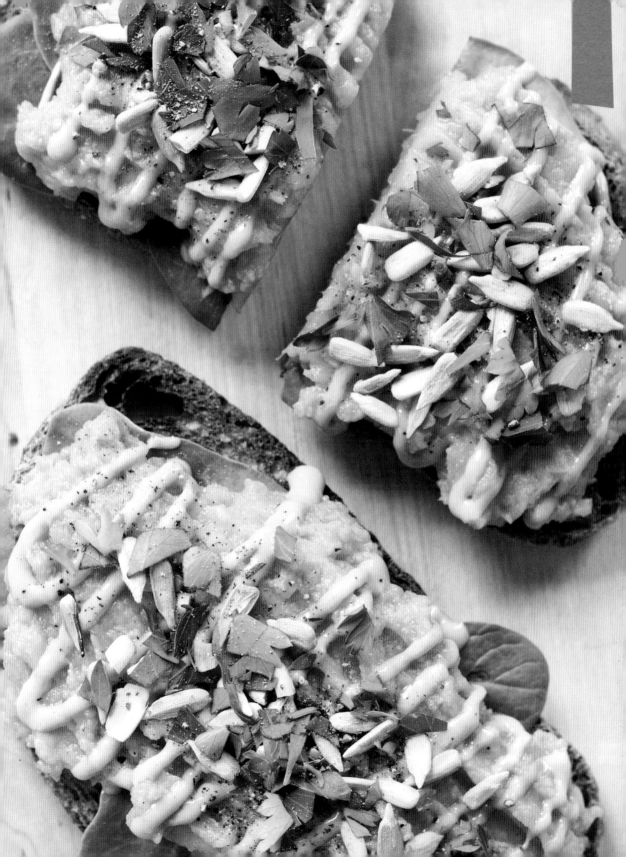

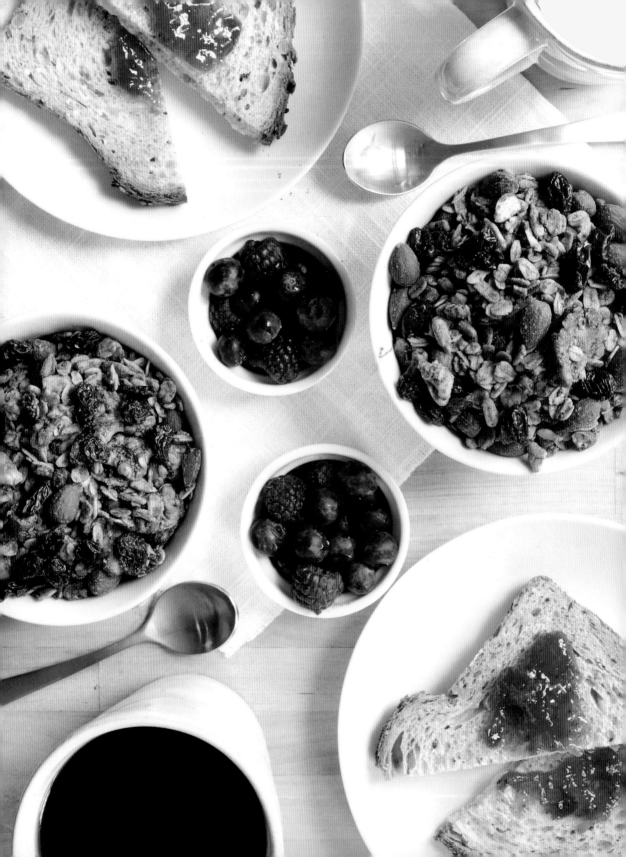

FILL-YOUR-BELLY
nutty GRANOLA

TOTAL TIME: 40 MINUTES   **ACTIVE TIME:** 10 MINUTES   **MAKES:** 8 SERVINGS

Store-bought granola is often filled with sugar and other ingredients that are less than amazing to kick off your day with. This version is tastier than any kind you can buy, plus the ingredients provide the perfect morning fuel.

DRY
2 cups rolled oats
½ cup walnuts, roughly
   chopped
½ cup almonds, roughly
   chopped
¼ cup sunflower seeds
2 tablespoons ground flaxseed
2 tablespoons chia seeds
1 tablespoon ground cinnamon
¼ teaspoon salt
2 tablespoons coconut sugar
   (optional)*

WET
½ cup creamy peanut butter
½ cup maple syrup
¼ cup coconut oil
1 tablespoon vanilla extract

ADD-IN
½ cup raisins and/or dried
   cranberries

1. Preheat the oven to 325°F.

2. In a large bowl, whisk the dry ingredients together.

3. In a small saucepan over low heat, combine the wet ingredients and heat them, stirring until smooth (3–4 minutes). Pour the mixture into the bowl with the dry ingredients and stir until everything is mixed.

4. Use a spatula to spread the mixture out on a baking sheet. Bake for 15 minutes, then remove the baking sheet from the oven and use the spatula to mix the granola. Return to the oven and bake for another 15 minutes.

5. Remove from the oven, and let the granola cool completely, allowing it to crisp up. Add the raisins or cranberries and transfer to an airtight container.

NOTE: *Transitioning away from processed, sugar-loaded cereal? Add a little coconut sugar and this recipe will help you step away from the sugary store brands.*

PUMPKIN SPICE *granola*

TOTAL TIME: 40 MINUTES   **ACTIVE TIME:** 10 MINUTES   **MAKES:** 8 SERVINGS

Don't you just love how there's always a feeling of excitement in the air when the first crisp fall breeze arrives and the leaves begin changing color? Suddenly everything is warm and cozy—and pumpkin flavored! I can't resist the magic of this season and even my morning granola gets a fall makeover.

DRY
2 cups rolled oats
⅔ cup raw pumpkin seeds
½ cup mixed nuts, roughly chopped
2 tablespoons pumpkin pie spice
⅛ teaspoon salt
2 tablespoons coconut sugar (optional)*

WET
½ cup pumpkin puree
½ cup maple syrup
2 tablespoons coconut oil, melted
2 tablespoons vanilla extract

ADD-IN
½ cup raisins or dried cranberries

1. Preheat the oven to 325°F.

2. In a large bowl, whisk the dry ingredients together.

3. In a small bowl, combine the wet ingredients. Add the contents of the small bowl to the large bowl and stir thoroughly.

4. Use a spatula to spread the mixture out on a baking sheet. Bake for 15 minutes, then remove the baking sheet from the oven and use the spatula to mix the granola. Return to the oven and bake for another 15 minutes.

5. Remove from the oven, and let the granola cool completely, allowing it to crisp up. Add the raisins or cranberries and transfer to an airtight container.

NOTE: *If you're using this as a dessert or smoothie topping, opt to add the coconut sugar.*

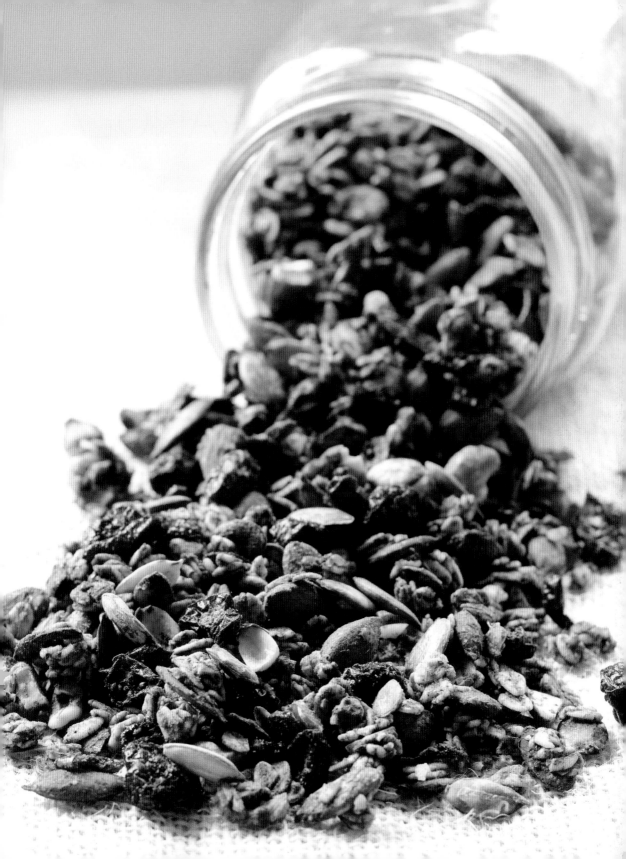

CHOCOLATE CHIP
banana bread GRANOLA

TOTAL TIME: 40 MINUTES   **ACTIVE TIME:** 10 MINUTES   **MAKES:** 8 SERVINGS

For a super-speedy breakfast or afternoon snack, throw a handful of this granola over some coconut yogurt and dig in.

DRY
2 cups rolled oats
½ cup pecans, roughly chopped
½ cup unsweetened coconut
  flakes
⅛ teaspoon salt

WET
1 ripe medium banana, mashed
¼ cup maple syrup
2 tablespoons coconut oil,
  melted
1 tablespoon vanilla extract

ADD-IN
½ cup chocolate chips

1. Preheat the oven to 325°F.

2. In a large bowl, whisk the dry ingredients together.

3. In a small bowl, combine the wet ingredients. Add the contents of the small bowl to the large bowl and stir thoroughly.

4. Use a spatula to spread the mixture out on a baking sheet. Bake for 15 minutes, then remove from the oven and use the spatula to mix the granola. Return to the oven and bake for another 15–20 minutes, until golden.

5. Remove from the oven, and let the granola cool completely, allowing it to crisp up. Add the chocolate chips and transfer to an airtight container.

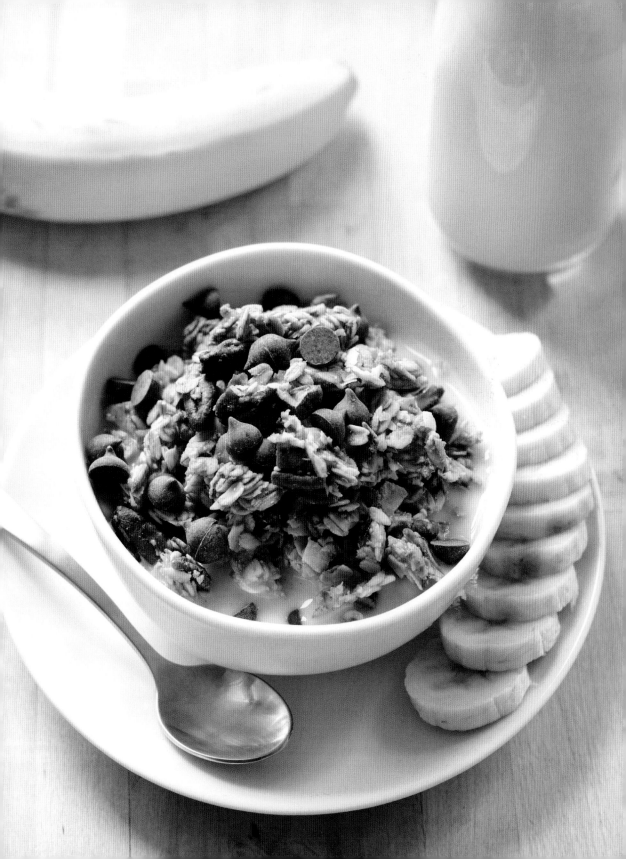

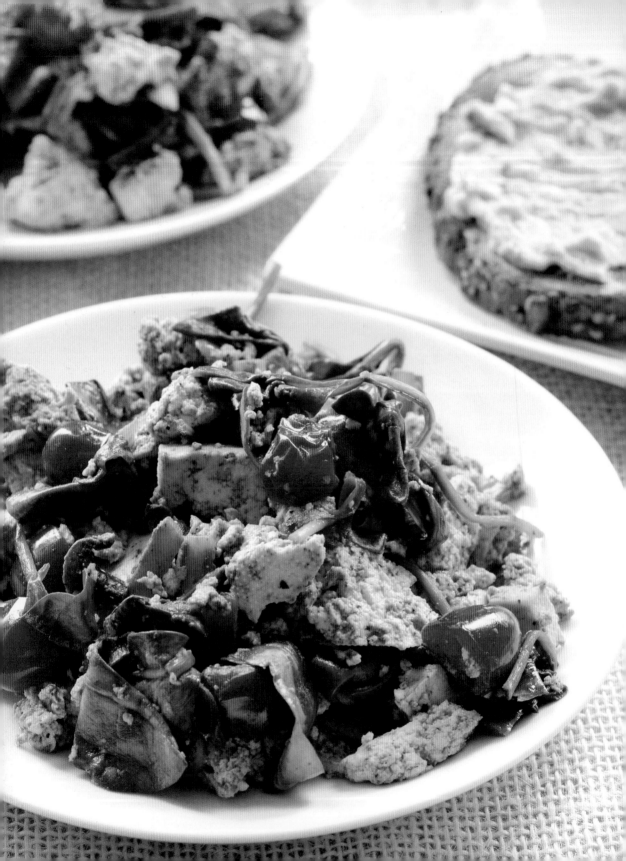

classic TOFU SCRAMBLE

TOTAL TIME: 15 MINUTES (PLUS TIME FOR PRESSING TOFU)   **MAKES:** 4 SERVINGS

For years, I loved ordering tofu scrambles at restaurants but could never make them taste as good at home. After many attempts, I eventually came up with this super-easy, restaurant-rivaling recipe that's perfect for brunch.

1 (14-ounce) package firm tofu
1 tablespoon olive oil
1 small red onion, diced
1 clove garlic, minced
1 cup sliced button or cremini mushrooms
2 cups packed baby spinach
1 cup cherry tomatoes, sliced in half
4 teaspoons tamari
2 tablespoons nutritional yeast
½ teaspoon ground turmeric
½ teaspoon paprika
Salt and black pepper, to taste

1. Cut the tofu into 1-inch slices. On a cutting board, layer the slices of tofu between paper towels or clean dishcloths. Place a heavy item (a teakettle filled with water works great) on top (or use a tofu press if you've got one). Let the tofu sit for at least 30 minutes (or overnight in the refrigerator for extra-amazing texture). This will remove the excess water from the tofu and give the scramble a better texture.

2. Heat the olive oil in a pan over medium heat. Add the onion, garlic, and mushrooms and cook for 5 minutes, stirring occasionally. Add the spinach and cherry tomatoes and cook for about 2 more minutes, until the spinach wilts.

3. Use your hands to crumble the tofu slices into the pan. Add the tamari, nutritional yeast, turmeric, paprika, salt, and pepper. Stir until everything is combined, and cook for another 3–5 minutes, until the mixture is heated through.

4. Transfer to plates and enjoy.

southwestern
TOFU SCRAMBLE

⊕ **TOTAL TIME:** 15 MINUTES (PLUS TIME FOR PRESSING TOFU) **MAKES:** 4 SERVINGS

Even though it's in the breakfast chapter, I often make this scramble when I need a great, easy weeknight dinner. If you're feeling wild, serve it with a scoop of Strawberry Mango Salsa (see page 144) on top.

SCRAMBLE
1 (14-ounce) package firm tofu
1 tablespoon olive oil
1 small red onion, diced
2 cloves garlic, minced
1 red bell pepper, sliced
1 cup cooked black beans
4 teaspoons tamari
2 tablespoons nutritional yeast
½ teaspoon ground turmeric
½ teaspoon paprika
Salt and black pepper, to taste

SERVE WITH
Avocado slices or guacamole
Salsa
Cashew Sour Cream (see
    page 226) or store-bought
    vegan sour cream
Chopped fresh cilantro
Tortilla chips

1. Cut the tofu into 1-inch slices. On a cutting board, layer the slices of tofu between paper towels or clean dishcloths. Place a heavy item (a teakettle filled with water works great) on top (or use a tofu press if you've got one). Let the tofu sit for at least 30 minutes (or overnight in the refrigerator for extra-amazing texture). This will remove the excess water from the tofu and give the scramble a better texture.

2. Heat the olive oil in a pan over medium heat. Add the onion and garlic and cook for 2 minutes. Add the bell pepper and cook for another 3 minutes, stirring occasionally.

3. Use your hands to crumble the tofu slices into the pan. Add the black beans, tamari, nutritional yeast, turmeric, paprika, salt, and pepper. Stir and cook for another 3–5 minutes, until everything is heated through.

4. Transfer to plates and top with the avocado or guacamole, salsa, **Cashew Sour Cream**, and cilantro. Serve with tortilla chips.

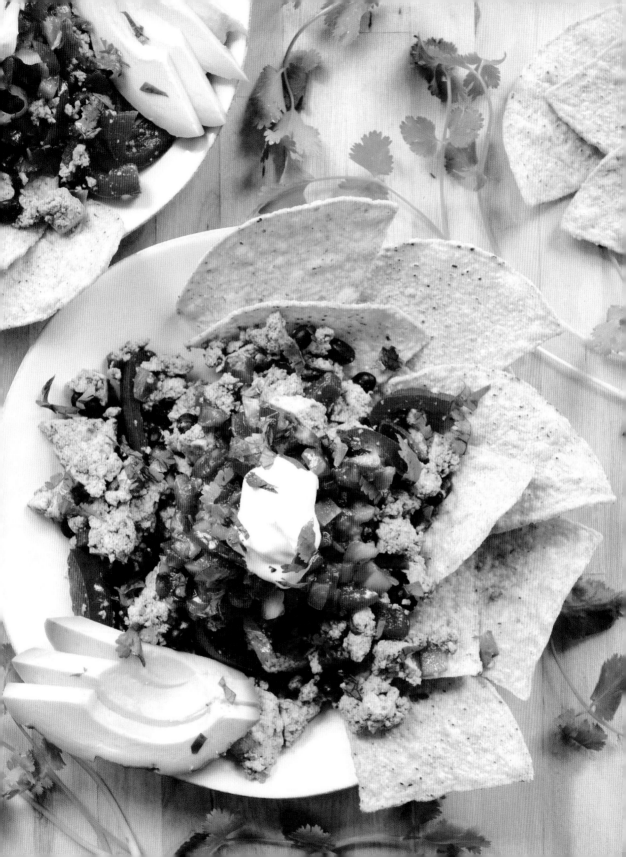

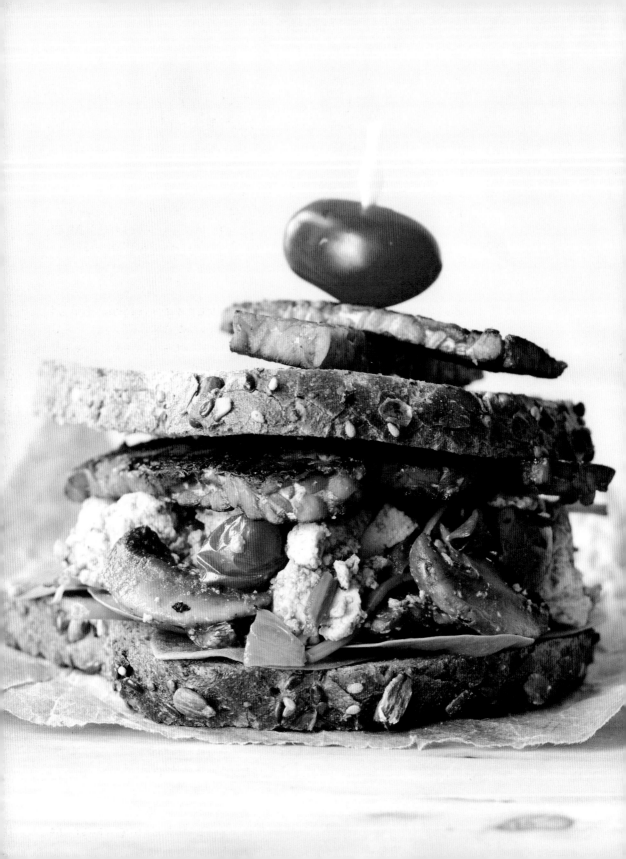

ULTIMATE *breakfast* *scramble* SANDWICH

⊕ **TOTAL TIME:** 5 MINUTES **MAKES:** 4 SANDWICHES

In my early twenties, I could stay out as late as I wanted, drink as much cheap wine as I wanted, and still wake up and go to work without a hangover. These days, if I have more than a glass and a half of wine at dinner, I need a gallon of green juice and a hearty breakfast to get my engine started the next day. This sandwich is my go-to for those kinds of mornings.

SANDWICHES
8 slices of bread (bagels
   or English muffins are
   great too)
1 cup packed baby spinach
1 batch Classic Tofu Scramble
   (see page 55)
1 batch Tempeh Bacon (see
   page 231)

ADD-ON OPTIONS
½ cup shredded vegan cheese
1 avocado, sliced
2 tablespoons ketchup
Hot sauce, to taste

1. Toast the bread.

2. To assemble the sandwiches, place 4 slices of the bread on plates and layer the spinach over each.

3. Spoon the Classic Tofu Scramble on top of the spinach, and add 3–4 slices of the Tempeh Bacon to each sandwich.

4. Top with any or all of the add-ons, then place the remaining 4 slices of bread on top and enjoy.

no-bake TRAIL MIX BARS

TOTAL TIME: 15 MINUTES (PLUS TIME FOR CHILLING) **MAKES:** 12–14 BARS

I'll never understand it, but my husband is one of those people who can completely forget to eat lunch. If I miss a meal (or even my afternoon snack), you better believe I'm constantly thinking about it—plus complaining about it to anyone within earshot. Getting "hangry" (hungry plus angry) is no joke for me, so I always keep ready-to-go snacks around. These protein-filled bars are one of my secret weapons for fighting "hanger."

DRY
½ cup chopped raw almonds
½ cup chopped raw walnuts
½ cup raw pumpkin seeds
½ cup raw sunflower seeds
½ cup shredded coconut
¼ cup raisins
¼ cup dried cranberries
⅛ teaspoon salt

WET
½ cup brown rice syrup
½ cup creamy peanut butter
2 tablespoons coconut oil
1 teaspoon vanilla extract

1. Line a baking sheet with parchment paper.

2. In a large bowl, whisk the dry ingredients together.

3. In a small saucepan over medium-low heat, cook the wet ingredients. Stir continuously until everything has melted, about 5 minutes.

4. Pour the melted mixture into the bowl of dry ingredients, and stir until thoroughly mixed.

5. Spoon the mixture onto the baking sheet, and use a spatula to press it firmly into a rectangle about ¾ inch thick.

6. Place the baking sheet in the refrigerator until it's completely cool, at least 1 hour. Remove and use a knife to slice into bars. Wrap the bars individually and store them in a large airtight container.

NOTE: *The bars will fall apart if they are left out for too long, so keep them in the fridge until you're ready to enjoy them.*

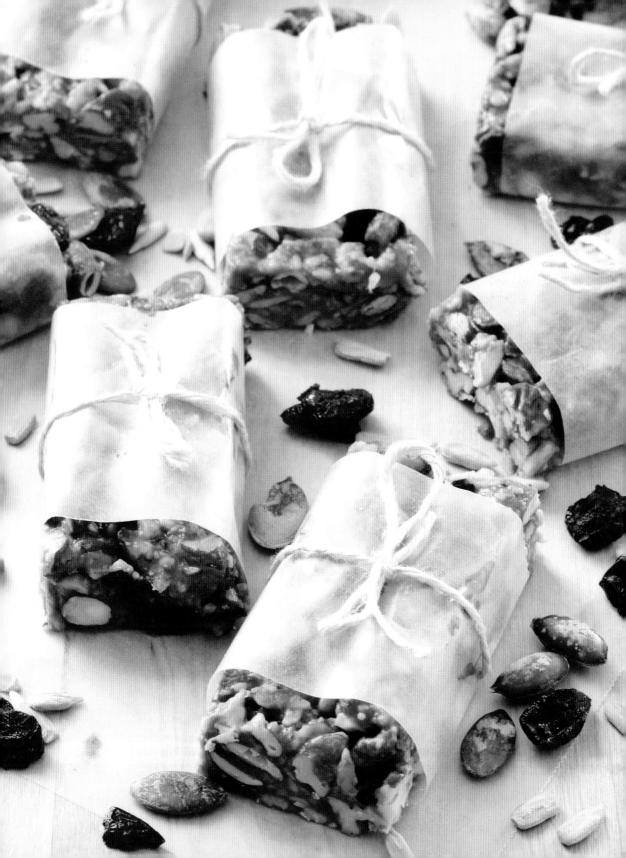

KALE & *oatmeal* BREAKFAST BARS

TOTAL TIME: 40 MINUTES   **ACTIVE TIME:** 15 MINUTES   **MAKES:** 8–10 BARS

One of the things I love about having a blog dedicated to colorful cooking is finding ways to sneak greens into unexpected recipes. Even though they are filled with kale, these bars are closer to a cookie than a salad.

DRY
1 cup rolled oats
½ cup chopped mixed nuts
¼ cup shredded coconut
2 tablespoons chia seeds
2 tablespoons ground flaxseed
1 tablespoon ground cinnamon
¼ teaspoon salt

WET
1 ripe medium banana, mashed
½ cup nondairy milk
¼ cup coconut oil, melted
3 tablespoons maple syrup
2 teaspoons vanilla extract

FOLD-INS
1 cup finely shredded kale
⅓ cup raisins

1. Preheat the oven to 325°F. Grease an 8-by-8-inch glass baking dish.

2. In a large bowl, whisk the dry ingredients together.

3. In a small bowl, stir the wet ingredients together until smooth. Add the contents of the small bowl to the large bowl and mix until thoroughly combined. Fold in the kale and raisins. Transfer the batter to the baking dish and use a spatula to spread it out evenly.

4. Bake for 25 minutes. Remove the baking dish from the oven and let it cool completely. Using a knife, slice into bars and store in an airtight container.

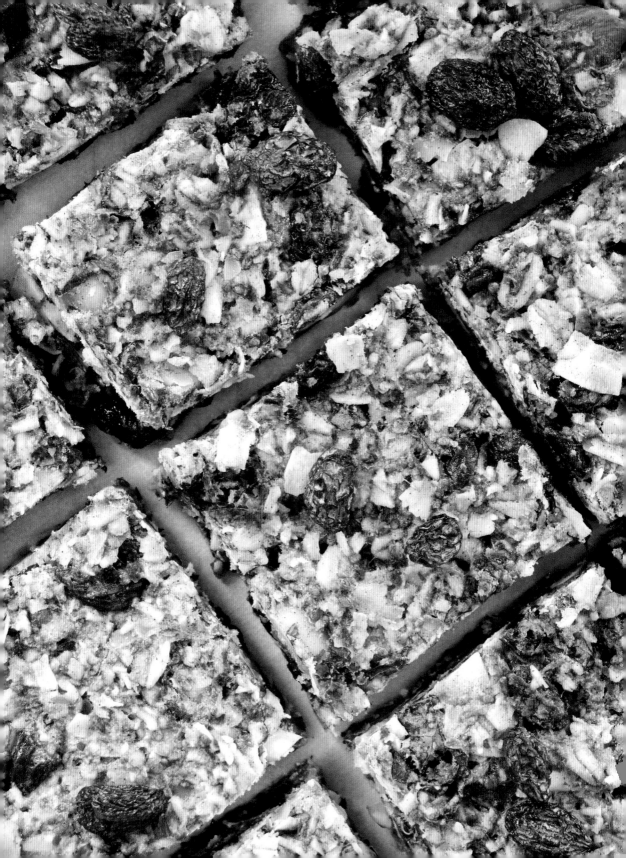

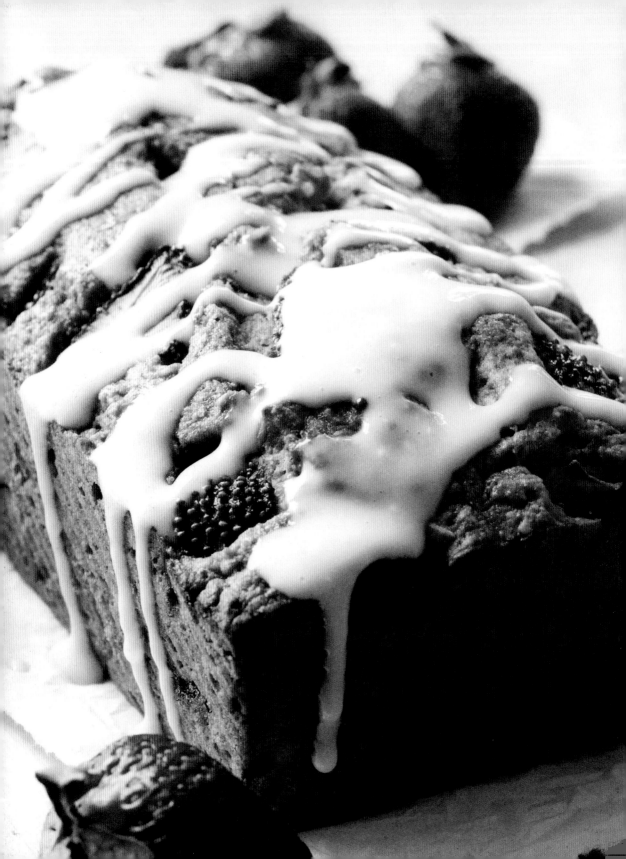

STRAWBERRY LOAF *with* CREAM CHEESE GLAZE

TOTAL TIME: 1 HOUR **ACTIVE TIME:** 15 MINUTES **MAKES:** 1 LOAF (ABOUT 8 SERVINGS)

I love this loaf served fresh with its cream cheese glaze, but it's also lovely sliced, toasted, and spread with vegan or coconut butter.

DRY
2 cups spelt flour
1 cup rolled oats
1 tablespoon baking powder
2 teaspoons ground cinnamon
¼ teaspoon salt

WET
½ cup coconut oil, melted
½ cup maple syrup
1 cup nondairy milk
Juice of 1 lemon
1 tablespoon vanilla extract

FOLD-IN
1 cup chopped strawberries

TOPPING
1 tablespoon coconut sugar

CREAM CHEESE GLAZE
¼ cup vegan cream cheese
3 tablespoons maple syrup

1. Preheat the oven to 375°F. Grease a 9-by-5-inch loaf pan.

2. In a large bowl, whisk the dry ingredients together.

3. In a small bowl, stir the wet ingredients together. Add the contents of the small bowl to the large and stir until thoroughly combined. Fold in the strawberries.

4. Transfer the batter to the loaf pan and use a spatula to spread it out evenly. Sprinkle the coconut sugar on top.

5. Bake for about 45 minutes, until the top is golden and crisp. Remove from the oven and let cool.

6. While the loaf cools, prepare the cream cheese glaze by stirring the cream cheese and maple syrup together in a small bowl until smooth. When the loaf is cool enough to handle, remove it from the pan and drizzle about one-quarter of the glaze on top. Save the rest to add a dollop to each slice when serving.

APPLE CINNAMON
crumb MUFFINS

TOTAL TIME: 40 MINUTES **ACTIVE TIME:** 15 MINUTES **MAKES:** 14 MUFFINS

Just like your favorite coffee-shop muffins, these babies are sweet, filling, and perfect alongside a cup of coffee. However, unlike most coffee-shop muffins, they're made of totally wholesome ingredients.

DRY
2 cups spelt flour
1 cup rolled oats
1 tablespoon baking powder
1 tablespoon ground cinnamon
⅛ teaspoon salt

WET
½ cup coconut oil, melted
½ cup maple syrup
1 cup nondairy milk
2 teaspoons vanilla extract

FOLD-IN
2 apples, peeled and diced

CRUMB TOPPING
1 cup spelt flour
⅓ cup coconut sugar
½ cup coconut oil, melted
1 tablespoon ground cinnamon
Dash of salt

DRIZZLE
⅓ cup coconut butter, melted

1. Preheat the oven to 350°F. Grease a muffin tin or line it with baking cups. (Since this recipe yields 14 muffins, you may want to prep two tins!)

2. In a large bowl, whisk the dry ingredients together.

3. In a small bowl, stir the wet ingredients together. Add the contents of the small bowl to the large bowl, and stir until thoroughly mixed. Fold in the apples.

4. Spoon the batter into the muffin tin wells (or baking cups) until they are three-quarters full.

5. Prepare the crumb topping by stirring the ingredients together in a medium bowl. Press the crumb topping over the batter in the baking cups until they are almost full.

6. Bake for 25 minutes. Remove and let the muffins cool completely. Drizzle the coconut butter on top and enjoy.

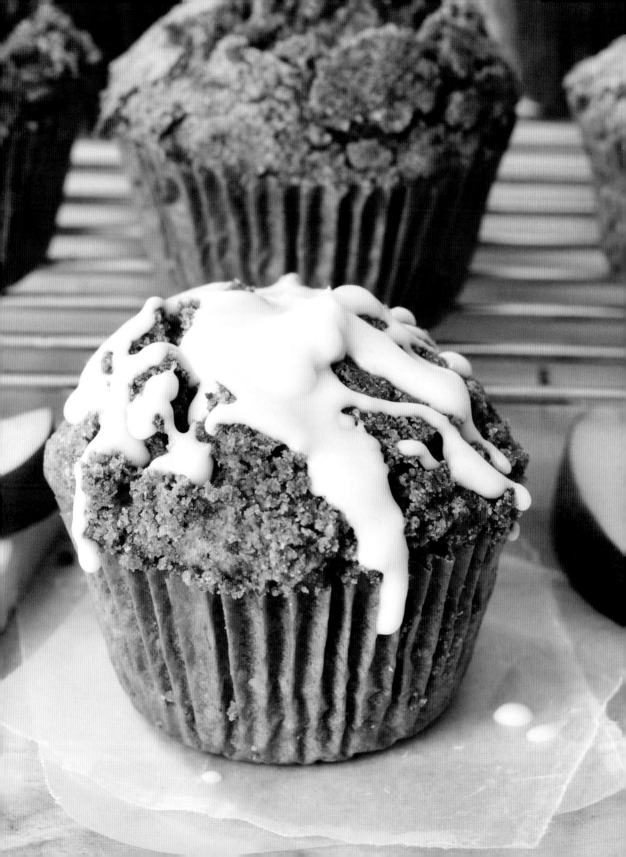

BLUEBERRY *basil* LEMON MUFFINS

TOTAL TIME: 40 MINUTES   **ACTIVE TIME:** 15 MINUTES   **MAKES:** 12 MUFFINS

This was another "pregnant lady" concoction of mine, and I was delighted to find out that it was still delicious after my little girl arrived and all my crazy cravings subsided. The addition of basil to these muffins makes the flavor a little funky—in the best way possible!

DRY
2 cups spelt flour
1 cup rolled oats
1 tablespoon baking powder
⅛ teaspoon salt

WET
½ cup coconut oil, melted
½ cup maple syrup
1 cup nondairy milk
2 teaspoons vanilla extract
Juice of 1 lemon
1 tablespoon grated
    lemon zest

FOLD-INS
1¼ cups blueberries (fresh
    or frozen)
2 tablespoons chopped
    fresh basil

SPRINKLE
1 tablespoon coconut sugar
Dash of salt

1. Preheat the oven to 350°F. Grease a muffin tin or line it with baking cups.

2. In a large bowl, whisk the dry ingredients together.

3. In a small bowl, stir the wet ingredients together. Add the contents of the small bowl to the large bowl, and stir until thoroughly mixed. Fold in the blueberries and basil.

4. Spoon the batter into the muffin tin wells (or baking cups) until they are just shy of full. Sprinkle the coconut sugar and salt on top.

5. Bake for 25 minutes. Remove and let the muffins cool before enjoying.

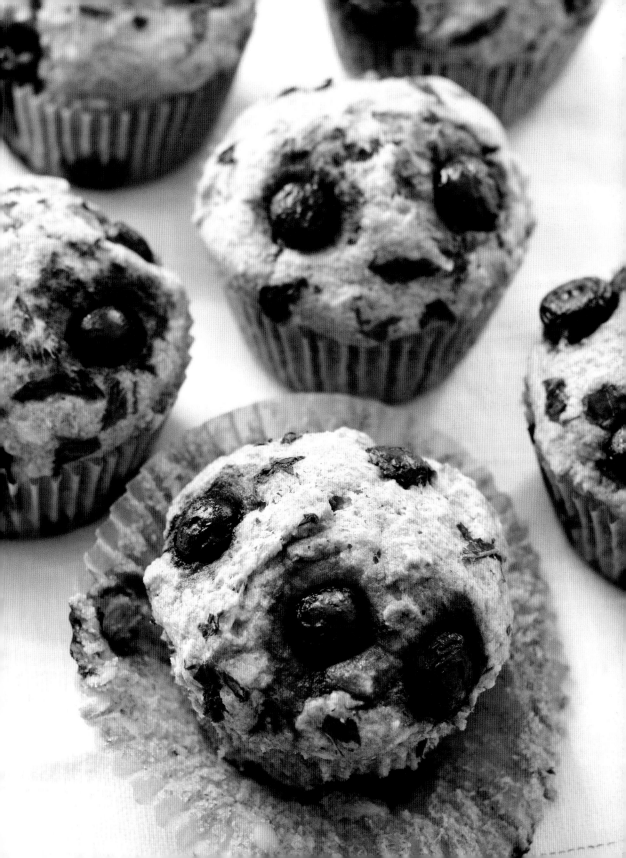

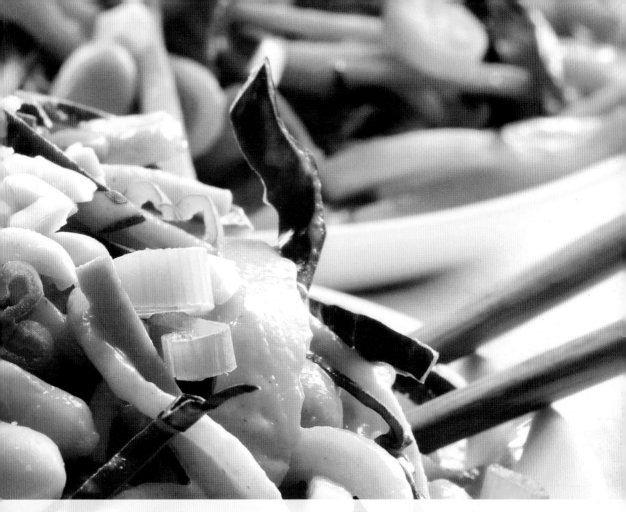

salads

EASY *kale* SALAD

TOTAL TIME: 10 MINUTES   MAKES: 4 SERVINGS

This is the perfect side dish to accompany just about any meal. Use this recipe as a starting point, then throw in whatever ingredients call your name. I like to use this salad as a bed of greens for veggie burgers or a filling in sandwiches, or serve it with veggies piled high on top.

DRESSING
Juice of ½ lemon
2 tablespoons olive oil
1 tablespoon tamari
1 tablespoon tahini, plus
   extra for drizzling
1 teaspoon maple syrup
Salt and black pepper, to taste

SALAD BASE
1 bunch kale, shredded

ADD-ONS
1 avocado, sliced
1 cup cherry tomatoes, sliced
   in half
1 red onion, sliced
¼ cup sunflower seeds

1. Stir the dressing ingredients together in a large bowl.

2. Add the kale. Use your hands to massage the dressing into the kale until it wilts, about 2 minutes. Top with the add-ons (or include your own additions) and toss. Transfer to plates and serve.

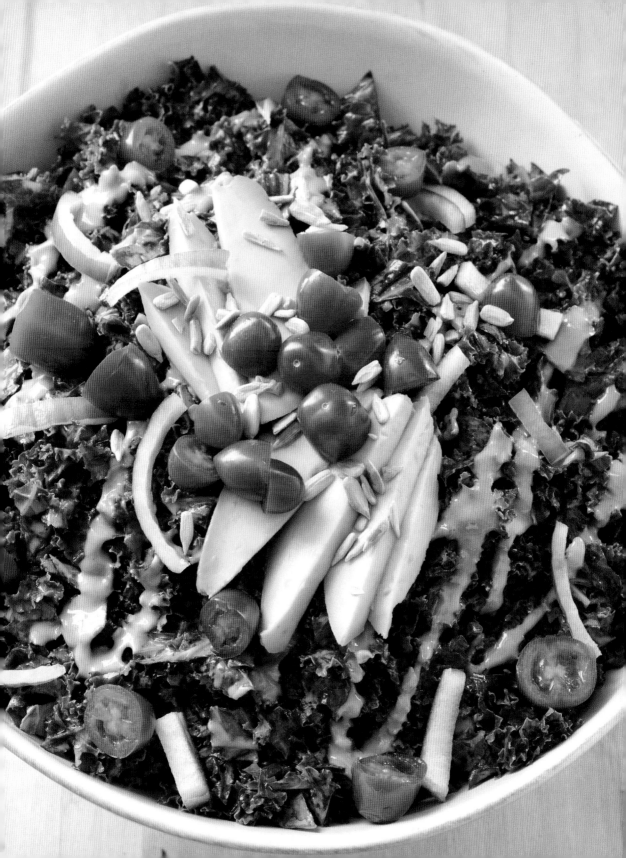

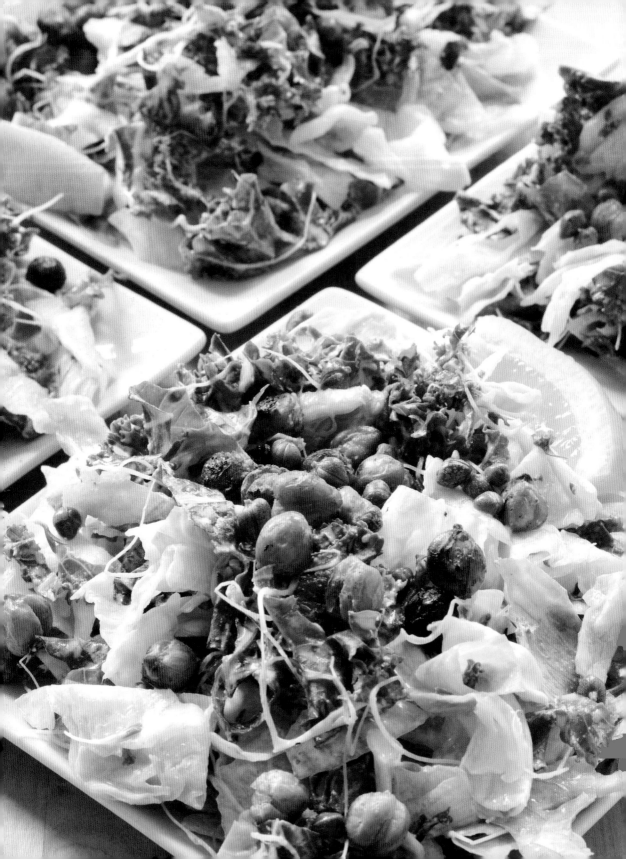

CRISPY CHICKPEA & KALE *caesar salad*

⊕ **TOTAL TIME:** 40 MINUTES   **ACTIVE TIME:** 20 MINUTES   **MAKES:** 4–6 SERVINGS

My family, especially my dad, used to be huge fans of those Caesar salad-in-a-bag kits that are 90 percent croutons and 10 percent wilted brown lettuce. The ingredients in this version are 100 percent good for you, and even my dad agrees it tastes way better than our old staple.

CRISPY CHICKPEAS

1½ cups cooked chickpeas (or one 15-ounce can, rinsed and drained)

1 tablespoon olive oil

½ teaspoon garlic powder

½ teaspoon smoked paprika

Salt and black pepper, to taste

SALAD

1 small head romaine lettuce, chopped

1 small bunch kale, shredded

1 cup sprouts

2 tablespoons capers

1 batch Caesar Dressing (see page 235)

Salt and black pepper, to taste

1 lemon, cut into wedges

1. To prepare the crispy chickpeas, preheat the oven to 425°F. Toss all the ingredients in a small bowl, until the chickpeas are completely coated. Spread them out on a baking sheet. Bake for 15 minutes, then remove from the oven and use a spatula to mix the chickpeas. Return them to the oven and bake for 10 more minutes. Remove and let them cool.

2. In a large bowl, combine the lettuce, kale, sprouts, and capers. Add the crispy chickpeas, and toss with the Caesar Dressing. Transfer to plates, sprinkle with salt and pepper, and garnish with the lemon wedges.

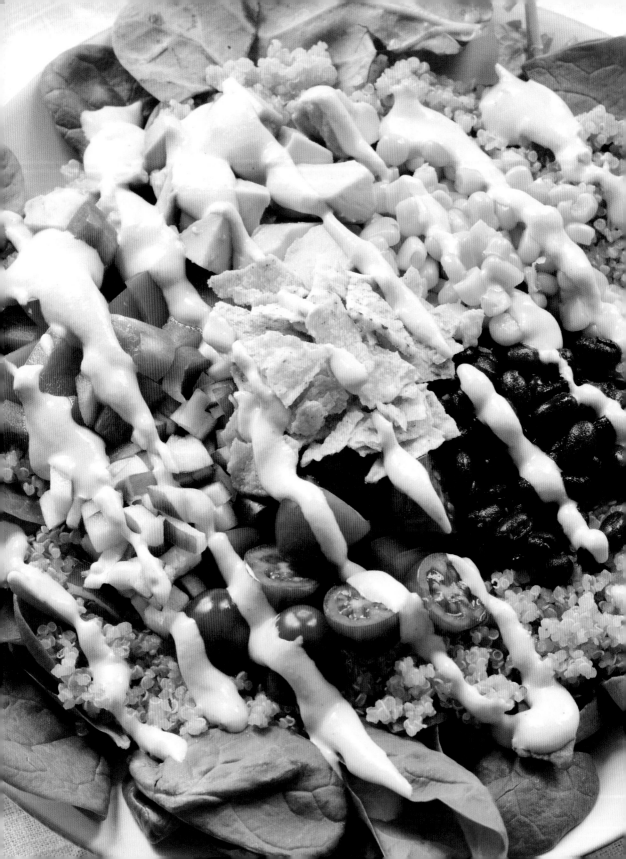

southwestern SALAD WITH GREEN CASHEW RANCH DRESSING

⊕ **TOTAL TIME:** 10 MINUTES **MAKES:** 4–6 SERVINGS

Hearty quinoa and a cashew-based dressing elevate this dish from "just a salad" to a totally filling lunch or dinner.

4 cups packed baby spinach
1 batch Quinoa (see page 228)
1½ cups cooked black beans
  (or one 15-ounce can,
  rinsed and drained)
1 cup cherry tomatoes,
  chopped
1 cup corn kernels
1 red bell pepper, chopped
1 small red onion, chopped
2 avocados, chopped
1 handful crushed tortilla chips
1 batch Green Cashew Ranch
  Dressing (see page 234)
Salt and black pepper, to taste

1. Put the spinach in a large bowl, and layer the Quinoa, black beans, cherry tomatoes, corn, bell pepper, onion, avocados, and tortilla chips on top.

2. Drizzle on the Green Cashew Ranch Dressing, and sprinkle salt and pepper on top. Transfer to plates and serve.

SHREDDED *brussels* SLAW

TOTAL TIME: 15 MINUTES   MAKES: 4 SERVINGS

This slaw is the perfect spotlight-stealing side dish to go with any entrée. If you find Brussels sprouts, broccoli, and cabbage to be a bit bitter, let the slaw sit in the fridge with the dressing on it for half an hour or so before enjoying.

DRESSING
Juice of 1 lemon
2 tablespoons olive oil
1 tablespoon balsamic vinegar
1 tablespoon maple syrup

SLAW
1½ cups shredded Brussels
   sprouts
1½ cups shredded broccoli
1½ cups shredded red cabbage
1 cup shredded carrots
½ cup raisins
½ cup slivered almonds
Salt and black pepper, to taste

1. In a small bowl, stir the dressing ingredients together.

2. In a large bowl, toss the slaw ingredients together. Stir in the dressing, and season with salt and pepper.

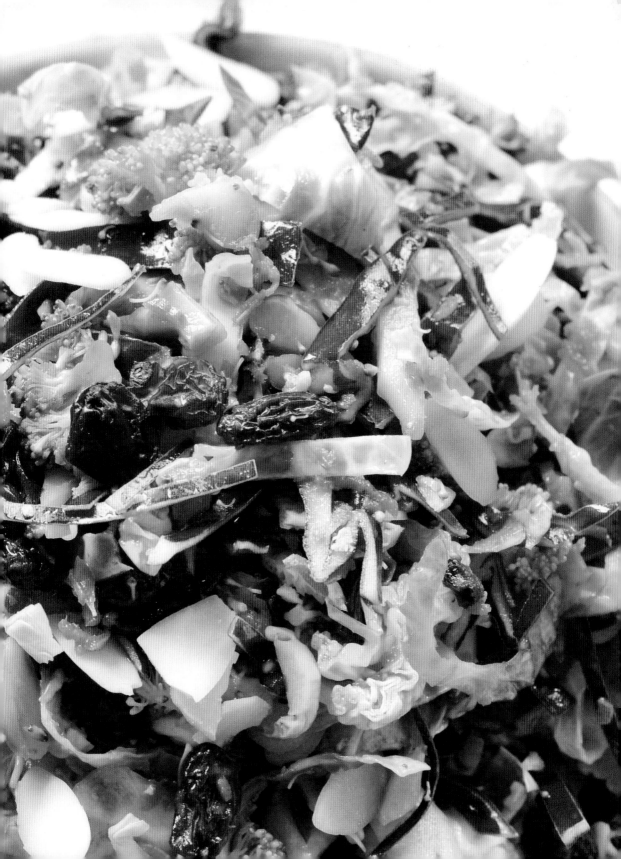

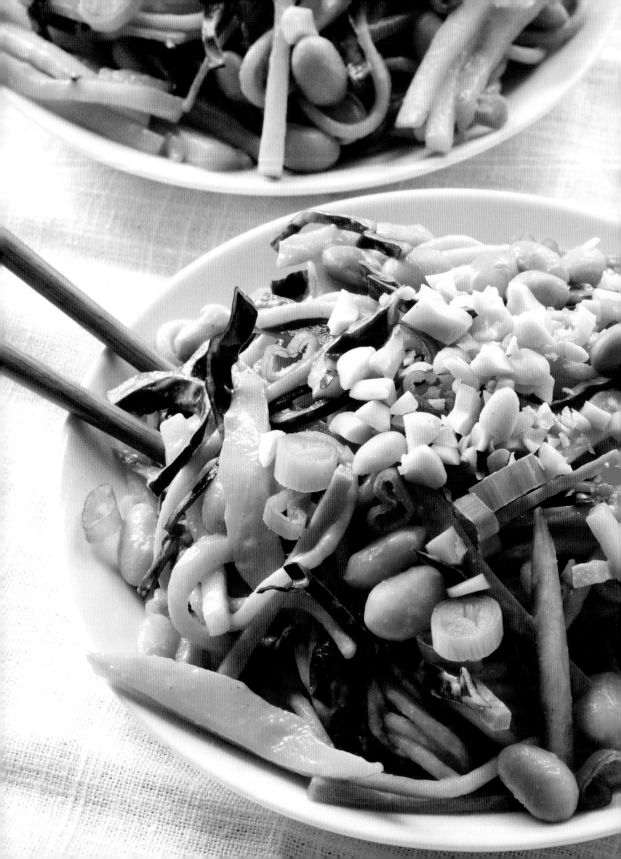

edamame PEANUT NOODLE SALAD

⊕ **TOTAL TIME:** 15 MINUTES **MAKES:** 4 SERVINGS

This easy meal is filled with tons of color, texture, and flavor. It makes a great quick lunch or a perfect cool dinner on hot summer nights when you can't bear to turn on the oven.

4 servings of soba or brown rice noodles, uncooked
2 cups shelled edamame
1 cup thinly sliced carrot
1 cup thinly sliced cucumber
1 cup thinly sliced cabbage
1 mango, thinly sliced
1 batch Peanut Sauce (see page 236)
2 green onions, chopped
¼ cup chopped peanuts

1. Prepare the noodles according to the instructions on the package. Rinse the noodles in cold water to cool, then transfer them to a large bowl.

2. Add the edamame, carrots, cucumber, cabbage, and mango, and toss with the Peanut Sauce.

3. Transfer to plates and top with the green onions and peanuts.

MEDITERRANEAN *lentil* SALAD WITH TOFU FETA

⊕ **TOTAL TIME:** 20 MINUTES (PLUS TIME FOR MARINATING TOFU FETA)   **MAKES:** 4 SERVINGS

This salad is perfect for when you're craving something savory and filling that's still on the lighter side. I like to make a double batch of the tofu feta to add a sprinkle of savory protein to everything throughout the week.

TOFU FETA
¼ cup apple cider vinegar
Juice of 1 lemon
1 tablespoon miso paste
1 tablespoon tamari
2 tablespoons nutritional yeast
½ teaspoon garlic powder
½ teaspoon dried oregano
⅛ teaspoon black pepper
1 (14-ounce) package
    extra-firm tofu, cut into
    1-inch cubes

DRESSING
¼ cup olive oil
2 tablespoons balsamic vinegar
Juice of 1 lemon
1 teaspoon Dijon mustard
2 teaspoons maple syrup
1 clove garlic, minced
Salt and black pepper, to taste

SALAD
4 cups packed mixed greens
1 batch Lentils (see page 230),
    chilled
1 large tomato, diced
1 medium cucumber, diced
1 small red onion, sliced
¼ cup sliced olives
¼ cup chopped fresh parsley

1. To prepare the tofu feta, stir the apple cider vinegar, lemon juice, miso paste, tamari, nutritional yeast, garlic powder, oregano, and pepper together in a jar or storage container. Add the tofu and shake. Let the tofu sit in the refrigerator for at least 2 hours (overnight is great) to marinate, shaking a few times throughout.

2. To prepare the dressing, stir all the ingredients together in a small bowl.

3. To prepare the salad, combine all the ingredients in a large bowl. Toss with the dressing and top with the tofu feta. Serve immediately.

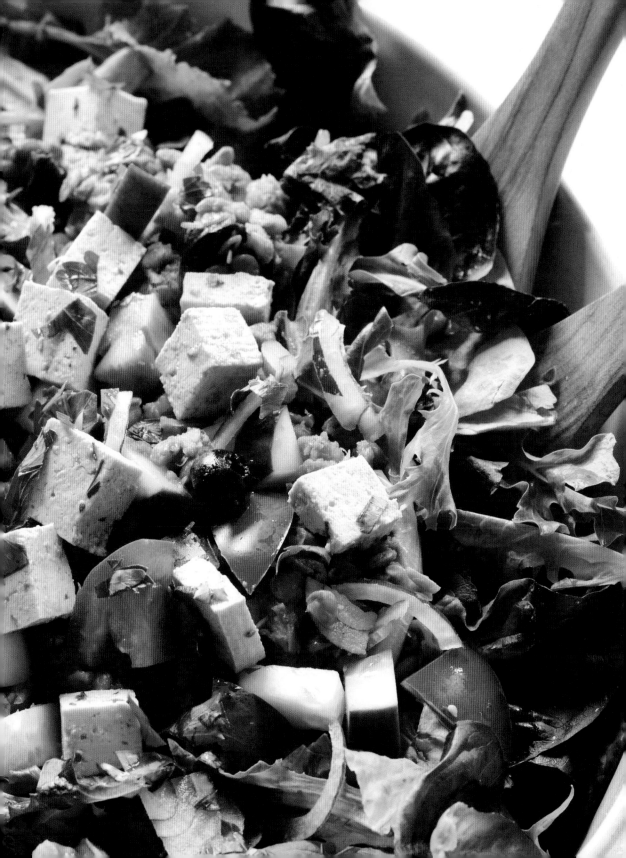

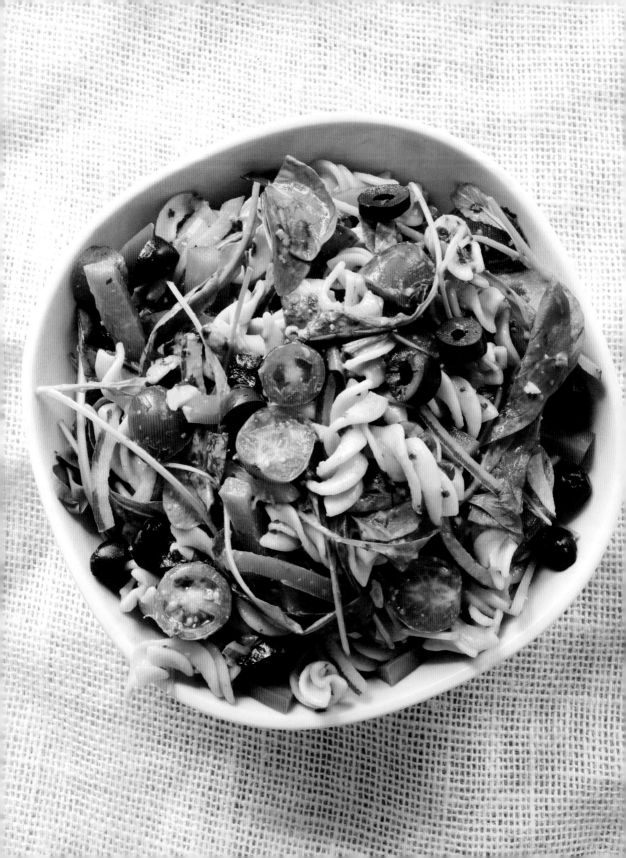

KALE & AVOCADO *pesto* PASTA SALAD

⊕ **TOTAL TIME:** 15 MINUTES   **MAKES:** 4 SERVINGS

I never understood pasta salad as a kid. Why would pasta exist if not to be smothered in marinara sauce and cheese? Decades later, I'm happy to report that I finally get it! Pasta salad can be light, fresh, and (best of all) bursting with colorful veggies. Double your batch of pesto and make Portobello & Potato Pesto Tacos *(see page 183) for dinner the next day.*

---

4 servings of fusilli pasta, uncooked
4 cups packed arugula
1 cup cherry tomatoes, chopped
1 small red onion, sliced
1 red bell pepper, sliced
¼ cup sliced Kalamata olives
1 batch Kale & Avocado Pesto (see page 236)
Salt and black pepper, to taste

1. Prepare the pasta according to the instructions on the package. Rinse the pasta in cold water to cool, then transfer it to a large bowl.

2. Add the arugula, cherry tomatoes, onion, bell pepper, olives, and Kale & Avocado Pesto to the bowl. Season with salt and pepper. Toss until mixed and enjoy immediately.

HUMMUS BOWL WITH
green tahini SAUCE

⊕ **TOTAL TIME:** 10 MINUTES   **MAKES:** 4 SERVINGS

I love this bowl as an easy-to-make lunch option. It's made of all my favorite ingredients—hummus is always my number-one midday fave.

1 bunch kale, chopped

1 avocado, sliced

1½ cups cooked chickpeas (or one 15-ounce can, rinsed and drained)

1 cucumber, sliced

1 cup cherry tomatoes, sliced in half

¼ cup Kalamata olives

2 green onions, chopped

½ cup hummus, store-bought or homemade (see pages 122–124)

1 batch Green Tahini Sauce (see page 238)

2 tablespoons chopped fresh parsley

Salt and black pepper, to taste

4 lemon wedges

1. Bring a pot of water to a boil over high heat. Put the kale in a steamer basket on top of the pot, cover, and steam for 2–3 minutes, until the kale is wilted. Divide the kale among individual serving bowls.

2. Layer the avocado, chickpeas, cucumber, cherry tomatoes, olives, and green onions over the kale. Add a scoop of the hummus in the center of each bowl.

3. Drizzle the Green Tahini Sauce over the bowls. Sprinkle the parsley, salt, and pepper on top and serve with the lemon wedges.

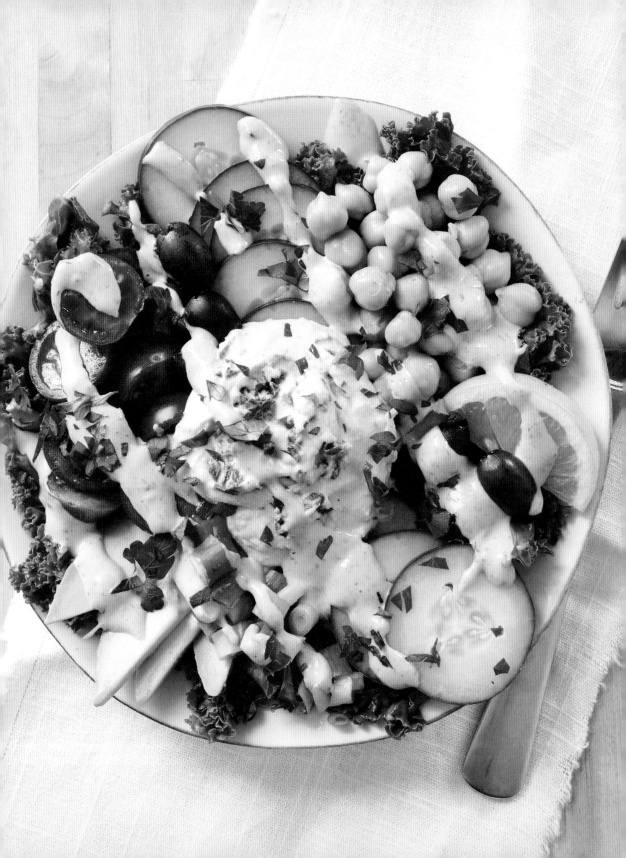

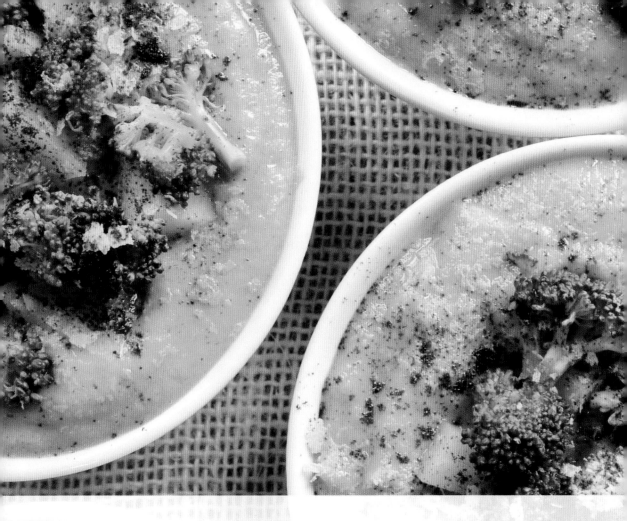

soup

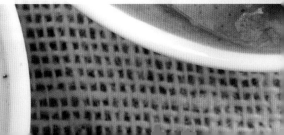

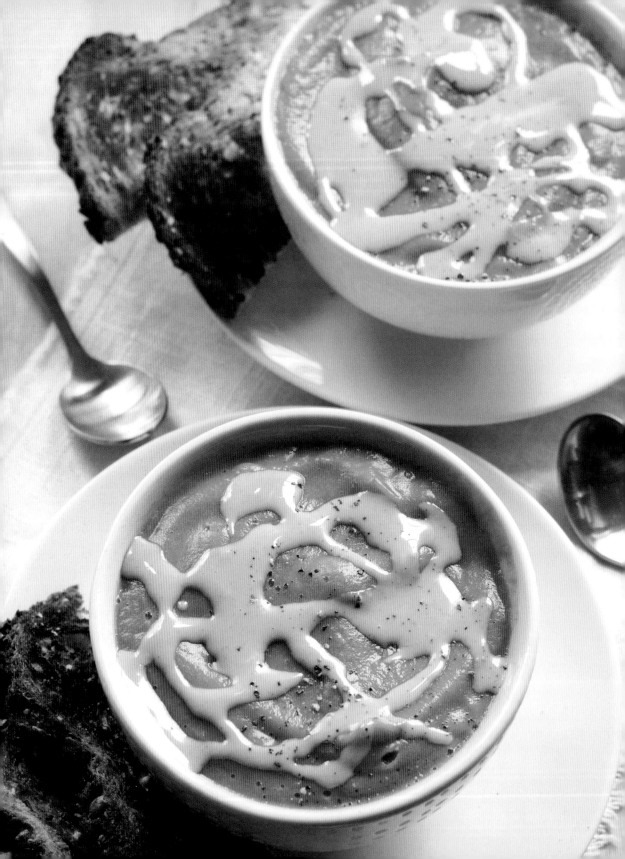

SWEET & SAVORY
sweet potato SOUP

TOTAL TIME: 30 MINUTES **ACTIVE TIME:** 15 MINUTES **MAKES:** 4 SERVINGS

This recipe has been a staple in my kitchen since I started cooking, and hardly a week goes by without a pot of it simmering on my stove. I like to double, triple, and quadruple it in the winter months so I always have an easy, warming meal or the perfect side dish in my fridge to knock out that down-to-your-bones chill.

1 tablespoon coconut oil
1 large onion, diced
4 cloves garlic, minced
3 cups vegetable broth
4 medium sweet potatoes, peeled and chopped into 1-inch pieces
1 tablespoon tamari
Salt and black pepper, to taste
¼ cup tahini

1. Heat the coconut oil in a large pot over medium-high heat. Add the onion and garlic and sauté until browned, about 7 minutes.

2. Add the vegetable broth and bring to a boil. Add the sweet potatoes and simmer until tender, about 15 minutes.

3. Turn off the heat and carefully transfer the mixture to a blender (let it sit for a few minutes if it is too hot to handle). Add the tamari, salt, and pepper, and blend until smooth.

4. Transfer to bowls, drizzle the tahini on top, and enjoy.

CREAMY, CHUNKY, *cheesy* BROCCOLI SOUP

TOTAL TIME: 35 MINUTES   ACTIVE TIME: 15 MINUTES   MAKES: 4 SERVINGS

White beans are the secret ingredient that makes this soup thick and creamy. I like to add Tempeh Bacon (see page 231) on top to make it extra hearty.

1 tablespoon olive oil
1 medium onion, diced
3 cloves garlic, minced
2 medium potatoes, peeled and cut into 1-inch pieces
2–3 cups vegetable broth
1 broccoli crown, broken into florets (about 2 cups)
1½ cups cooked white beans (or one 15-ounce can, rinsed and drained)
½ cup nutritional yeast, plus extra for sprinkling
1 tablespoon tamari
Salt and black pepper, to taste
1 teaspoon smoked paprika

1. In a large pot, heat the olive oil over medium-high heat. Add the onion and garlic and sauté until lightly browned, about 7 minutes.

2. Add the potatoes and enough vegetable broth to cover. Simmer for about 15 minutes, until tender.

3. Add the broccoli and cook for about 2 minutes, until the broccoli turns bright green. Scoop out 1 cup of the broccoli, potato, and onion mixture and set aside.

4. Turn off the heat and carefully transfer the contents of the pot to a blender (let it sit for a few minutes if it is too hot to handle). Add the white beans, nutritional yeast, and tamari, and blend until smooth.

5. Return the blended soup to the pot, heat to the desired warmth, and season with salt and pepper. Stir in the reserved broccoli, potato, and onions. Transfer to bowls and top with the smoked paprika and extra nutritional yeast.

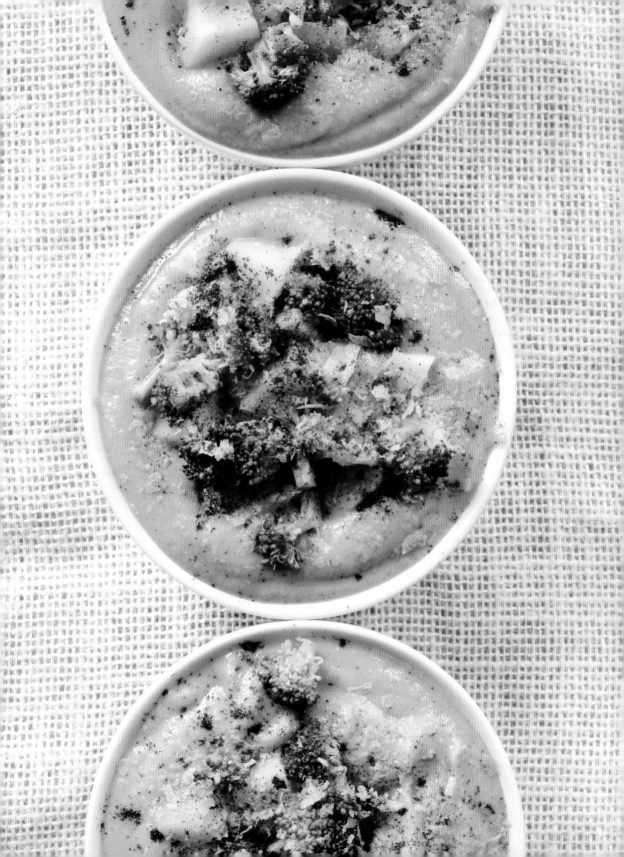

SWEET POTATO *chili*

⊕ **TOTAL TIME:** 1 HOUR 10 MINUTES   **ACTIVE TIME:** 30 MINUTES   **MAKES:** 4–6 SERVINGS

When I met my husband, his eating habits couldn't have been more different from mine. Living like a true New York City bachelor with a hearty appetite, he subsisted on takeout and giant burritos from the food truck on his block. This chili was one of the first recipes that got the "Wow, I guess you really don't need the meat!" reaction from him.

CHILI BASE

1 tablespoon coconut oil
1 medium onion, diced
3 cloves garlic, minced
1 (28-ounce) can crushed tomatoes
1 cup vegetable broth
3 medium sweet potatoes, peeled and cut into 1-inch chunks
1 cup chopped carrot
1 cup chopped celery
1½ cups cooked kidney beans (or one 15-ounce can, rinsed and drained)
1 tablespoon tamari
1 teaspoon cayenne pepper (or more for spicier chili)
1 teaspoon ground cumin
½ teaspoon paprika
½ teaspoon ground nutmeg
Salt and black pepper, to taste

SERVE WITH

1 batch Cashew Sour Cream (see page 226) or store-bought vegan sour cream
Shredded vegan cheddar cheese
2 green onions, chopped

1. Heat the coconut oil in a large pot over medium-high heat. Add the onion and garlic and sauté for about 7 minutes, until lightly browned.

2. Add the crushed tomatoes and vegetable broth and bring to a boil.

3. Add the sweet potatoes, carrots, and celery and simmer for about 40 minutes, until the sweet potatoes are very tender.

4. Stir in the kidney beans, tamari, cayenne pepper, cumin, paprika, nutmeg, salt, and pepper. Cook for a few more minutes, until everything is warm (simmer even longer for extra-thick chili). Serve with the Cashew Sour Cream, cheese, and green onions.

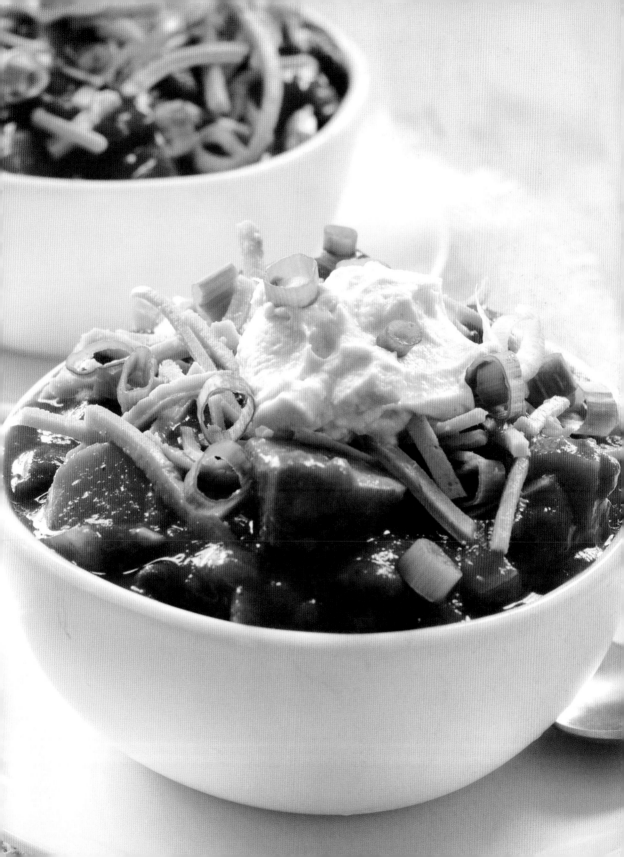

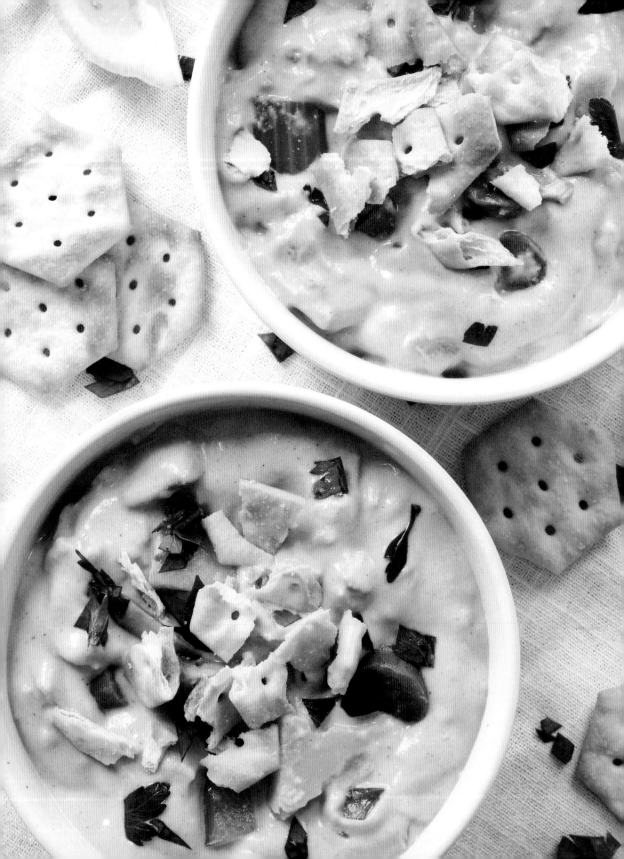

cauliflower CHOWDER

TOTAL TIME: 40 MINUTES (PLUS TIME FOR SOAKING CASHEWS)
ACTIVE TIME: 30 MINUTES   **MAKES:** 4–6 SERVINGS

Figuring out how to make things creamy without butter or milk was one of the biggest challenges in my early dairy-free days. Swapping in store-bought vegan versions of butter and milk can usually get the job done, but I think the real magic happens when a recipe relies completely on unprocessed ingredients. In this soup, cashews and cauliflower do the trick and come together to make it creamy-dreamy.

SOUP
1 medium cauliflower crown, broken into florets
2 tablespoons olive oil, divided
1 medium onion, diced
3 cloves garlic, minced
5 cups vegetable broth, divided
1½ cups chopped carrot
1½ cups chopped celery
1½ cups chopped button or cremini mushrooms
2 medium potatoes, peeled and chopped
1 cup raw cashews, soaked in water at least 4 hours
1 tablespoon miso paste
¼ cup nutritional yeast
1–2 tablespoons tamari, to taste
Salt and black pepper, to taste
Juice of 1 lemon

SERVE WITH
Lemon wedges
Chopped fresh parsley
Crackers

1. Preheat the oven to 425°F. In a bowl, toss the cauliflower with 1 tablespoon of the olive oil and spread it out on a baking sheet. Bake for 25 minutes, flipping halfway.

2. While the cauliflower bakes, heat the remaining 1 tablespoon olive oil over medium-high heat in a large pot. Add the onion and garlic and sauté for 5 minutes. Add 2 cups of the vegetable broth and bring to a boil. Add the carrot, celery, mushrooms, and potatoes and simmer for about 20 minutes, until everything is tender.

3. Drain and rinse the cashews. When the cauliflower is done baking, prepare the cauliflower cream by blending the cauliflower with the cashews, remaining 3 cups vegetable broth, and miso paste in a blender.

4. Stir the cauliflower cream into the pot. Add the nutritional yeast, tamari, salt, pepper, and lemon juice.

5. Transfer to bowls and serve with lemon wedges, parsley, and crackers.

loaded MISO NOODLE SOUP

TOTAL TIME: 20 MINUTES   **MAKES:** 4 SERVINGS

When I was little and I got sick, my mom would always make me noodle soup. (Remember the kind that came in a pouch?) Cuddling up under a blanket and slurping the broth from a mug was the most comforting thing in the world. This recipe gives me that same feeling, and I like to keep it in rotation for rainy nights and sick days.

4 servings of soba or brown rice noodles, uncooked

3 cups vegetable broth

3 cups water

1 cup julienned carrot*

1 cup julienned zucchini*

1 cup thinly sliced shiitake mushrooms

1 cup broccoli florets

3 tablespoons miso paste

1 (14-ounce) package firm tofu, cut into 1-inch cubes

¼ cup chopped green onions

1 sheet roasted nori seaweed, broken into pieces

1. Prepare the noodles according to the instructions on the package. Set them aside.

2. In a medium saucepan over high heat, bring the vegetable broth and water to a boil. Add the carrot, zucchini, mushrooms, and broccoli, reduce the heat, and simmer for 5 minutes.

3. Use a ladle to transfer 1 cup of broth to a small bowl. Use a fork to dissolve the miso paste into the broth, then return it to the pot. Add the tofu, green onions, and cooked noodles, then simmer for 1 more minute, until everything is warm.

4. Transfer to bowls and top with the nori seaweed.

NOTE: *"Julienned" means sliced into matchstick shapes.*

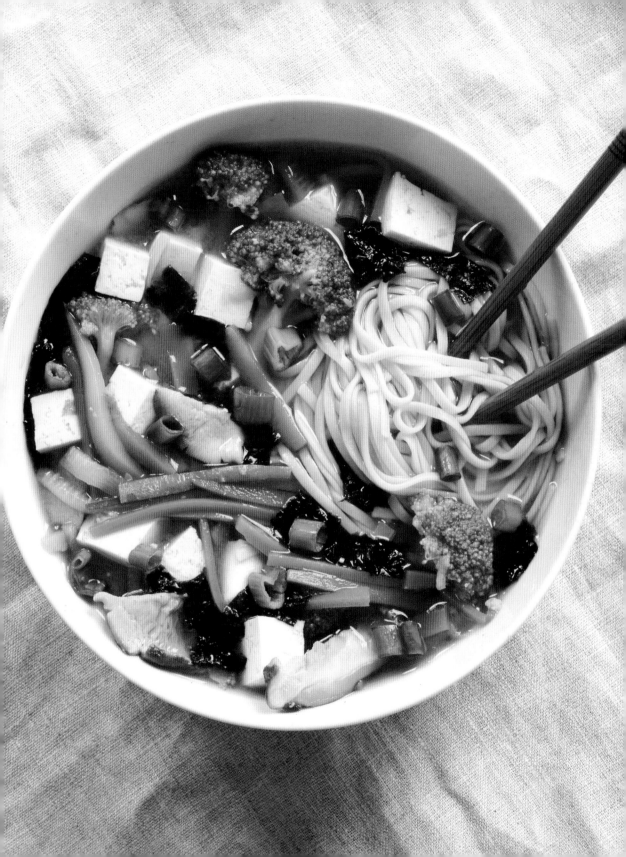

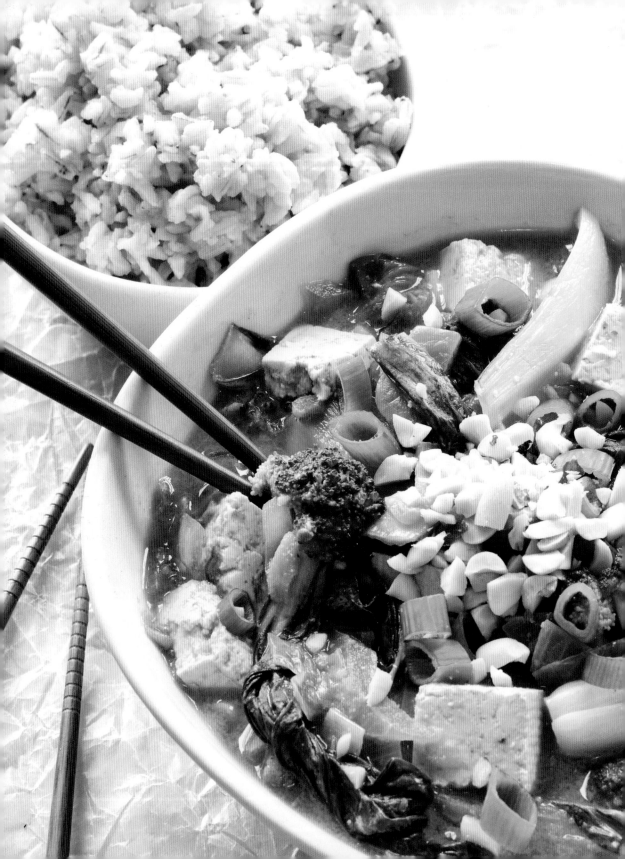

SPICY PEANUT & *kimchi* STEW

TOTAL TIME: 20 MINUTES **MAKES:** 4 SERVINGS

One cold night, my husband and I were playing the "But what do you want for dinner?" game, and we landed on the incredible stew from the Korean restaurant in our neighborhood. We weren't up for braving the cold and going out, so I came up with this version at home. If you like the tangy taste of kimchi, you'll love this nourishing soup. Make it extra filling by serving it over brown rice, quinoa, or noodles.

STEW
1 tablespoon coconut oil
1 medium onion, diced
2 cloves garlic, minced
2 cups vegetable broth
2 cups unsweetened
   nondairy milk*
1 cup kimchi, chopped*
6 tablespoons peanut butter
1 broccoli crown, broken into
   florets (about 2 cups)
4 heads baby bok choy, ends
   trimmed
1 (14-ounce) package firm
   tofu, cut into 1-inch cubes
Tamari, to taste

TOPPINGS
¼ cup chopped peanuts
2 green onions, chopped

1. In a large pot, heat the coconut oil over medium-high heat. Add the onion and garlic and sauté for 5 minutes.

2. Add the vegetable broth and nondairy milk and bring to a boil. Stir in the kimchi and peanut butter and simmer for 3 minutes, stirring occasionally.

3. Add the broccoli, bok choy, and tofu, then simmer for 5 more minutes. Add the tamari (the amount will vary depending on how salty your kimchi is).

4. Transfer to bowls and top with the peanuts and green onions.

NOTE: *For an extra creamy stew, use 1 (13½-ounce) can of full-fat coconut milk and ½ cup of another unsweetened nondairy milk of your choice.*

NOTE: *Store-bought kimchi often contains fish. Vegan options can usually be found at health-food stores; just be sure to check the label.*

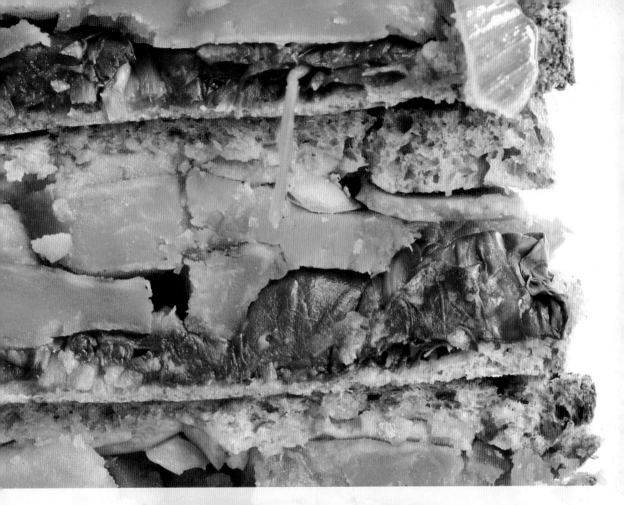

sandwiches

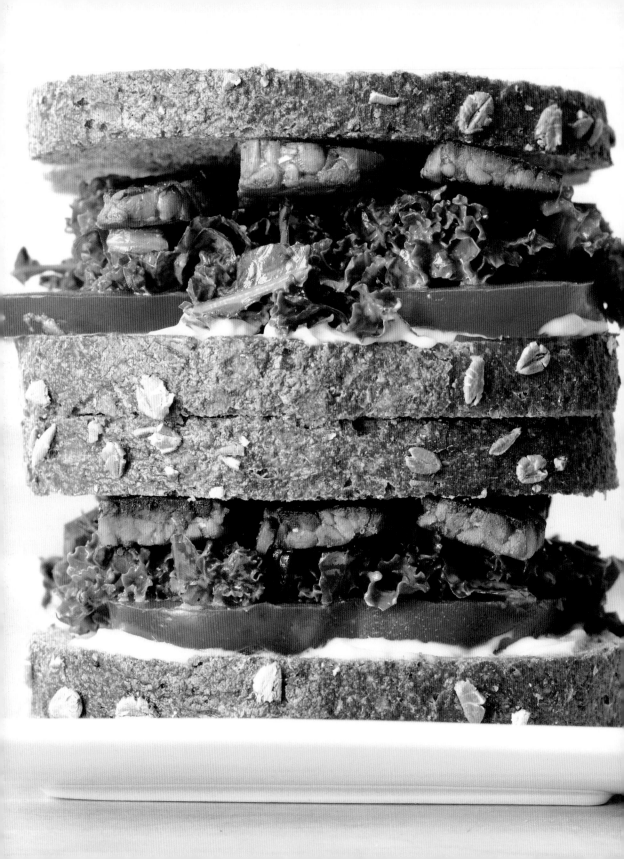

BKT (bacon kale tomato)

⊕ **TOTAL TIME:** 5 MINUTES **MAKES:** 4 SANDWICHES

Bye-bye BLT, hello BKT! The perfect balance between crunchy kale, creamy mayo, and hearty tempeh makes this sandwich a true upgrade.

8 slices of bread

2–3 tablespoons vegan mayo, store-bought or homemade (see page 224)

2–3 tablespoons mustard

2 medium tomatoes, sliced

½ batch Easy Kale Salad (see page 72)

1 batch Tempeh Bacon (see page 231)

Avocado slices (optional)

1. Toast the bread.

2. Spread the mayo on 4 slices of the bread. Spread the mustard on the other 4 slices.

3. To assemble the sandwiches, layer the tomatoes, **Easy Kale Salad**, **Tempeh Bacon**, and avocado (if using) on 4 of the slices of bread. Top with the other 4 bread slices.

4. Plate the sandwiches and enjoy immediately.

GRILLED REUBEN-*ish*

⊕ **TOTAL TIME:** 15 MINUTES **MAKES:** 4 SANDWICHES

I spent a good chunk of my childhood in Jewish-style delis in New York and South Florida (the unofficial Jewish grandparent headquarters) noshing on bagels and lox, tuna melts, and black-and-white cookies. This sandwich is inspired by a favorite I used to order with my bubbe (a.k.a. my gran).

8 slices of bread

1 batch Thousand Island Dressing (see page 235)

2 tablespoons Dijon mustard

1 handful mixed greens

1 batch Baked Tofu (see page 233), sliced

¼–½ cup sauerkraut

1 avocado, sliced

¼ cup sliced pickles

1. Spread 4 slices of the bread with the **Thousand Island Dressing.** Spread the mustard on the other 4 slices.

2. To assemble the sandwiches, layer the greens, **Baked Tofu,** sauerkraut, avocado, and pickles on 4 of the slices of bread. Top with the other 4 bread slices. Grill the sandwiches in a panini press* and enjoy warm.

NOTE: *I don't actually have a panini press, so I use an old electric grill that I rescued from my uncle's basement. You can also press the sandwich on the stove by heating it in a pan and placing something heavy (like another pan) on top.*

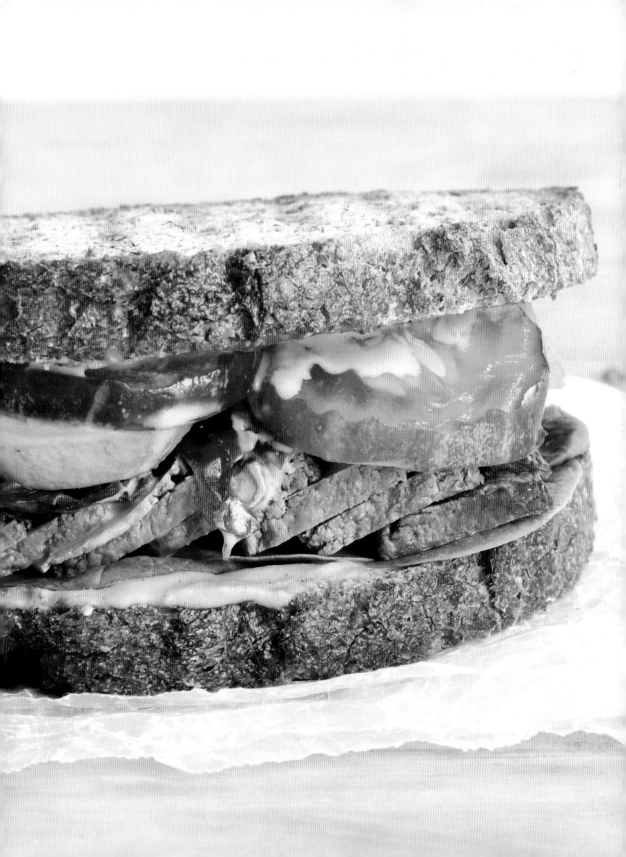

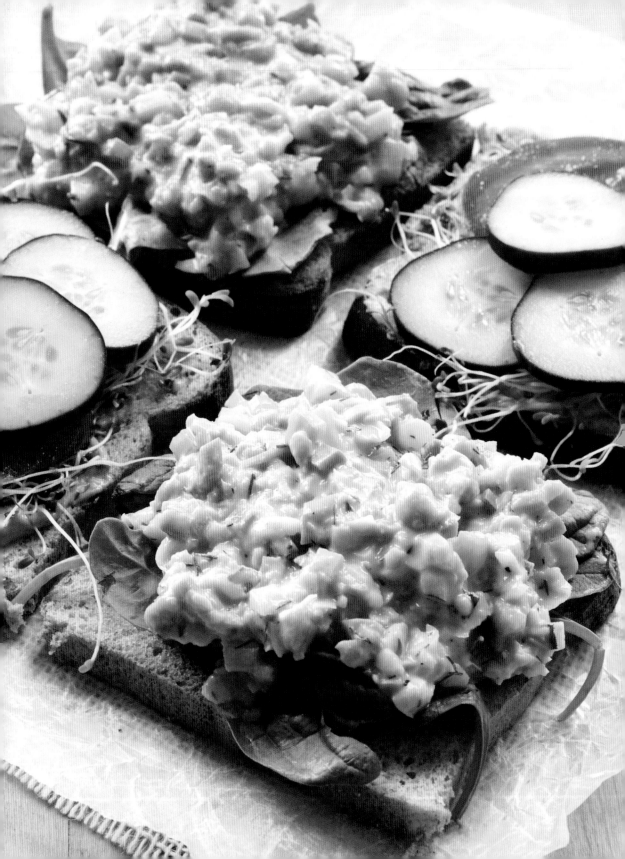

chickpea "TUNA" SALAD SANDWICH

⊕ **TOTAL TIME:** 15 MINUTES **MAKES:** 4 SANDWICHES

When I was growing up, tuna salad sandwiches were a staple in my house. Looking back, I think my family enjoyed the convenience of this sandwich more than the actual taste, but this updated version is both super-speedy and super-delicious.

CHICKPEA "TUNA" SALAD

1½ cups cooked chickpeas (or one 15-ounce can, rinsed and drained)

¼ cup diced carrot

¼ cup diced celery

2 tablespoons diced red onion

1 tablespoon chopped fresh dill

¼ cup vegan mayo, store-bought or homemade (see page 224)

Juice of ½ lemon

1 teaspoon apple cider vinegar

1 teaspoon pickle brine

Salt and black pepper, to taste

SANDWICHES

8 slices of bread

2 tablespoons Dijon mustard

1 handful greens

1 large tomato, sliced

1 cucumber, sliced

1 cup sprouts

1. To prepare the chickpea "tuna" salad, mash the chickpeas in a medium bowl with a potato masher or fork until a chunky texture is created. Stir in the carrot, celery, onion, dill, mayo, lemon juice, apple cider vinegar, pickle brine, salt, and pepper.

2. To assemble the sandwiches, spread 4 slices of the bread with the mustard, and layer them with the greens, tomato, cucumber, and sprouts. Add a heap of chickpea "tuna" salad and top with the other 4 bread slices.

PINEAPPLE & PEANUT SAUCE *tofu wrap*

⊕ **TOTAL TIME:** 10 MINUTES **MAKES:** 4 WRAPS

Isn't pineapple and peanut an oddly appealing flavor combination? This wrap is the perfect medley of sweet and savory flavor. My favorite wraps are brown rice tortillas, which you can usually find in the freezer section of health-food stores.

1 batch Peanut Sauce (see page 236)
4 large wraps*
1 batch Baked Tofu (see page 233), sliced
1 cup packed baby spinach
1 cup thinly sliced carrot
1 cup thinly sliced cabbage
1 cup sliced pineapple

1. To assemble the wraps, spread 1 tablespoon of the **Peanut Sauce** down the center of each wrap. Layer each wrap with the tofu, spinach, carrot, cabbage, and pineapple, and roll up each wrap. (Use a toothpick to secure the wraps.)

2. Serve with extra **Peanut Sauce** for dipping.

NOTE: *I prefer gluten-free brown rice wraps, which can usually be found in the freezer section of the grocery store.*

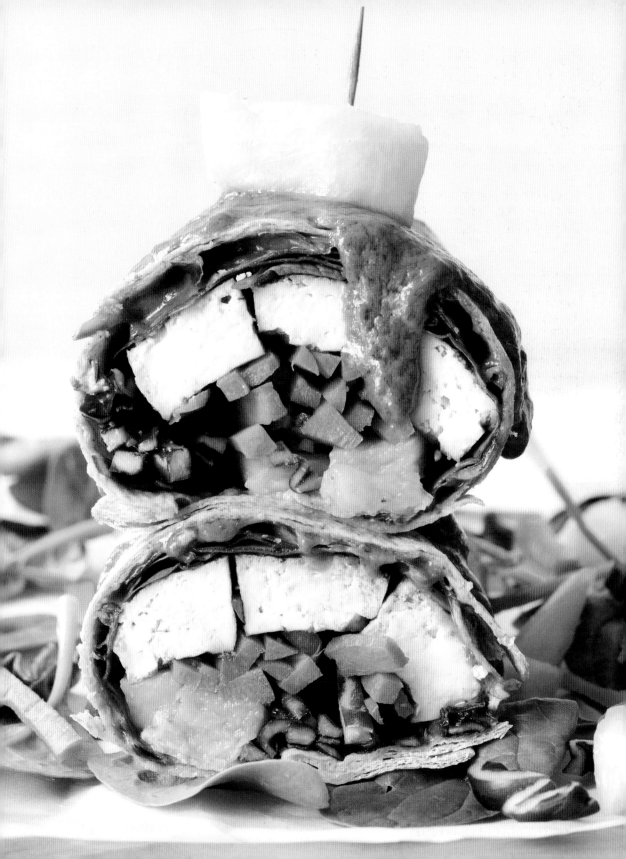

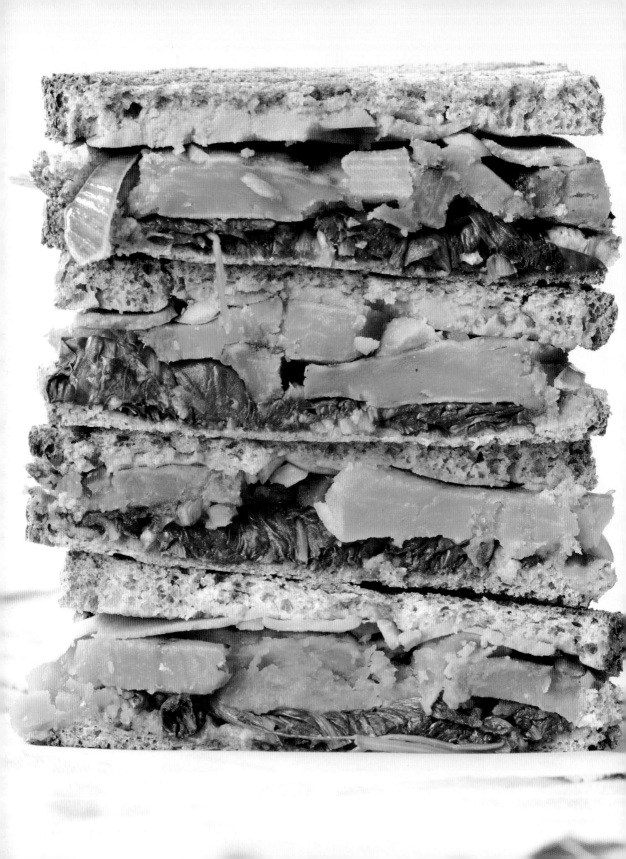

MAPLE-MUSTARD SQUASH *grilled cheese*

⊕ **TOTAL TIME**: 15 MINUTES   **MAKES**: 4 SANDWICHES

I originally came up with this recipe on the fly as a way to use up all the leftovers in my fridge in one meal, but it quickly became a fall and winter lunchtime go-to.

6 cups packed baby spinach
8 slices of bread
½ batch Maple-Mustard Sauce (see page 237)
½ batch Maple-Mustard Squash (see page 188)
1 small red onion, sliced
4 slices vegan cheddar cheese

1. Wilt the spinach by placing it in a pan with a splash of water over medium heat. Stir until wilted, about 2 minutes, and remove from the heat.

2. Spread 4 slices of the bread with the **Maple-Mustard Sauce**.

3. To assemble the sandwiches, layer the wilted spinach, **Maple-Mustard Squash**, onion, and cheese on 4 of the slices of bread. Top with the other 4 bread slices. Grill the sandwiches in a panini press* until the cheese melts and enjoy warm.

NOTE: *See the note about panini press alternatives in Grilled Reuben-ish (page 106).*

RAINBOW *beet* & *hummus* SANDWICH

⊕ **TOTAL TIME:** 10 MINUTES   **MAKES:** 4 SANDWICHES

Is it just me or does food taste better when it's arranged in rainbow order? Here's a delicious way to find out.

8 slices of bread
¼ cup Balsamic Beet Spread (see page 143)
¼ cup hummus, store-bought or homemade (see pages 122–124)
½ cup thinly sliced cabbage
1 handful baby spinach
1 avocado, sliced
½ cup thinly sliced carrot
½ cup thinly sliced yellow bell pepper
1 tomato, sliced

1. Spread 4 slices of the bread with the **Balsamic Beet Spread**. Spread the hummus on the other 4 slices.

2. To assemble the sandwiches, layer the cabbage, spinach, avocado, carrot, bell pepper, and tomato (in that order) over the slices that are spread with hummus. The result will be a beautiful rainbow effect. Top with the slices of bread that are covered with the **Balsamic Beet Spread**.

3. Place on plates and serve immediately.

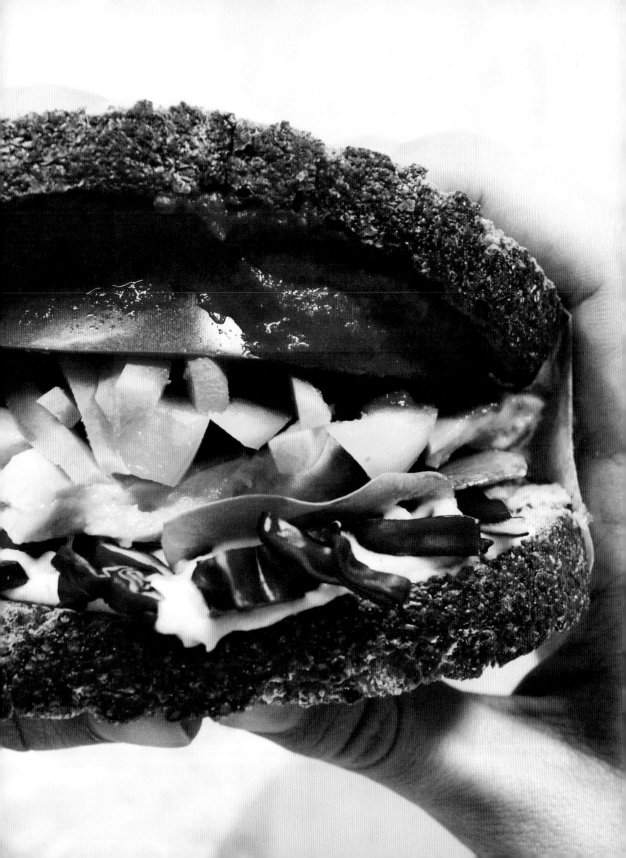

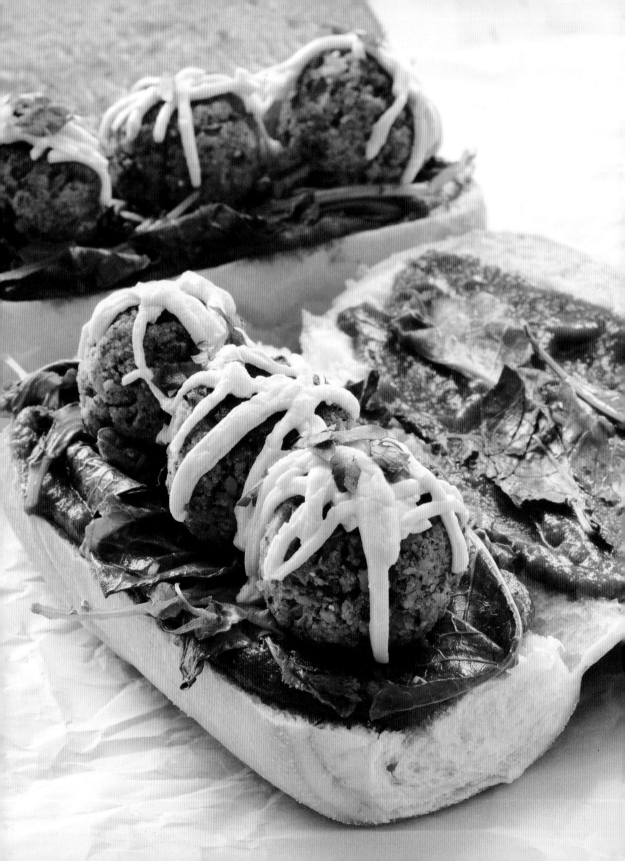

MEATBALL & *garlicky greens* SUB

It was a really big deal when a popular sandwich chain opened up near the neighborhood I grew up in. I can still remember my younger brother begging me to take him there to get meatball subs. In researching recipes for this book, I looked up the ingredients list on its website and— holy moly—there are ridiculous amounts of unpronounceable ingredients in those sandwiches. My updated version has all the warm and melty qualities we loved back in the day and none of the funky stuff.

1 batch Tempeh-Mushroom Meatballs (see page 157), leftover or freshly made

1 cup marinara sauce

1 tablespoon olive oil

2 cloves garlic, minced

4 cups packed greens of your choice (kale, spinach, Swiss chard, etc.)

4 rolls

½ cup shredded vegan mozzarella cheese (optional)

Salt and black pepper, to taste

1. If using leftover meatballs, preheat the oven to 400°F. Place the meatballs on a baking sheet and bake for 7–10 minutes, until warm.

2. Warm the marinara sauce in a small saucepan over low heat.

3. To prepare the garlicky greens, heat the olive oil in a pan over medium-high heat. Add the garlic and cook for 1 minute. Add the greens and stir until wilted, about 2 minutes. Remove from the heat.

4. To assemble the sandwiches, slice the rolls open. Spread the sauce on the bottom halves of the rolls, then top with the garlicky greens, cheese (if using), meatballs, salt and pepper, and top halves of the rolls. Enjoy warm.

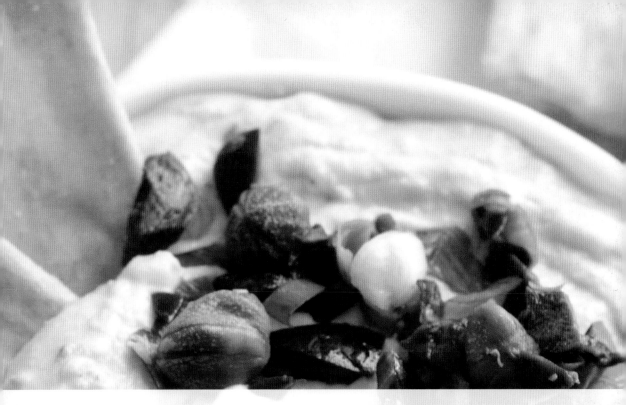

sides, snacks & appetizers

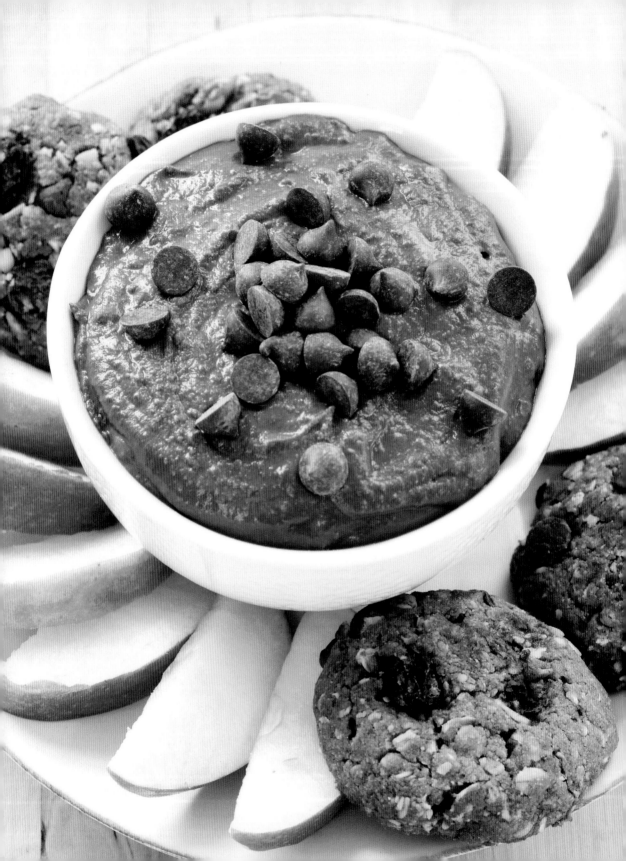

chocolate HUMMUS

TOTAL TIME: 10 MINUTES **MAKES:** 6 SERVINGS

I admit it—chocolate hummus sounds ultra-weird, and I was scared it would turn off my readers when I put this recipe up on my blog. I'm happy to say that I was wrong and I'm definitely not the only one who loves this sweet and savory dip. Enjoy it as a light, fresh snack with fruit slices, or get extra indulgent and spread it over cookies.

1½ cups cooked chickpeas (or one 15-ounce can, rinsed and drained)*
¼ cup creamy peanut butter
4 Medjool dates, pitted*
¼ cup cocoa powder
3 tablespoons maple syrup
2–3 tablespoons nondairy milk
1 teaspoon vanilla extract
Dash of salt
1 handful chocolate chips

SERVING OPTIONS
Apple slices
Banana slices
Cookies
Crackers

1. Combine the chickpeas, peanut butter, dates, cocoa powder, maple syrup, nondairy milk, vanilla extract, and salt in a blender or food processor and blend until smooth.

2. Transfer to a serving dish and sprinkle with the chocolate chips. Serve with fruit slices, cookies, crackers, or anything that sounds good.

NOTE: *For the creamiest, dreamiest hummus, peel off the skins from the chickpeas before blending. It takes a little bit of time, but you'll be rewarded with the smoothest hummus you've ever had.*

NOTE: *If you aren't using a high-speed blender, you may want to soften the dates by soaking them in hot water for 5 minutes so they blend smoothly.*

SUPER-SAVORY *hummus*

TOTAL TIME: 10 MINUTES **MAKES:** 6 SERVINGS

If you're all about the salty snacks and you like to pile on the olives and capers, add this hummus to your snack roster.

HUMMUS
1½ cups cooked chickpeas (or one 15-ounce can, rinsed and drained)*
¼ cup tahini
2 tablespoons olive oil
Juice of ½ lemon
2 cloves garlic, crushed
2 tablespoons water
Salt, to taste

ADD-INS
10 Kalamata olives, pitted and finely chopped
2 green onions, finely chopped
2 tablespoons capers, finely chopped

1. Combine all the hummus ingredients in a blender or food processor and blend until smooth.

2. Transfer to a serving bowl and stir in half of the olives, green onions, and capers. Sprinkle the other half on top.

NOTE: *For the creamiest, dreamiest hummus, peel off the skins from the chickpeas before blending. It takes a little bit of time, but you'll be rewarded with the smoothest hummus you've ever had.*

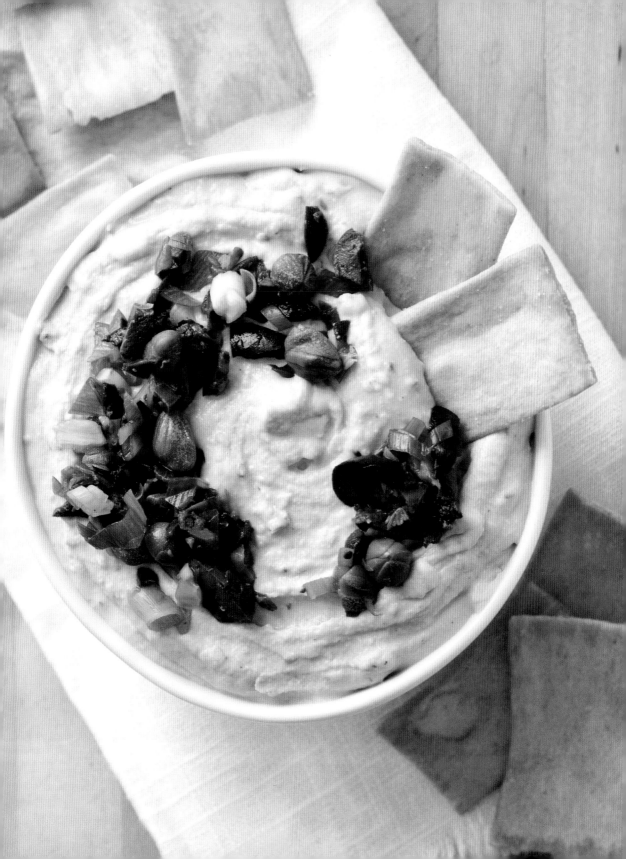

GREEN PARSLEY &
fresh lemon HUMMUS

TOTAL TIME: 10 MINUTES **MAKES:** 6 SERVINGS

This hummus is light, bright, and fresh tasting. I like it best served with raw veggies.

1½ cups cooked chickpeas (or one 15-ounce can, rinsed and drained)*

½ cup packed fresh parsley, plus extra for sprinkling

Juice of 1 lemon

¼ cup tahini

2 tablespoons olive oil

1 clove garlic, crushed

2 tablespoons water

Salt, to taste

1. Combine all the ingredients in a blender or food processor and blend until smooth.

2. Transfer to a serving bowl and sprinkle the extra parsley on top.

NOTE: *For the creamiest, dreamiest hummus, peel off the skins from the chickpeas before blending. It takes a little bit of time, but you'll be rewarded with the smoothest hummus you've ever had.*

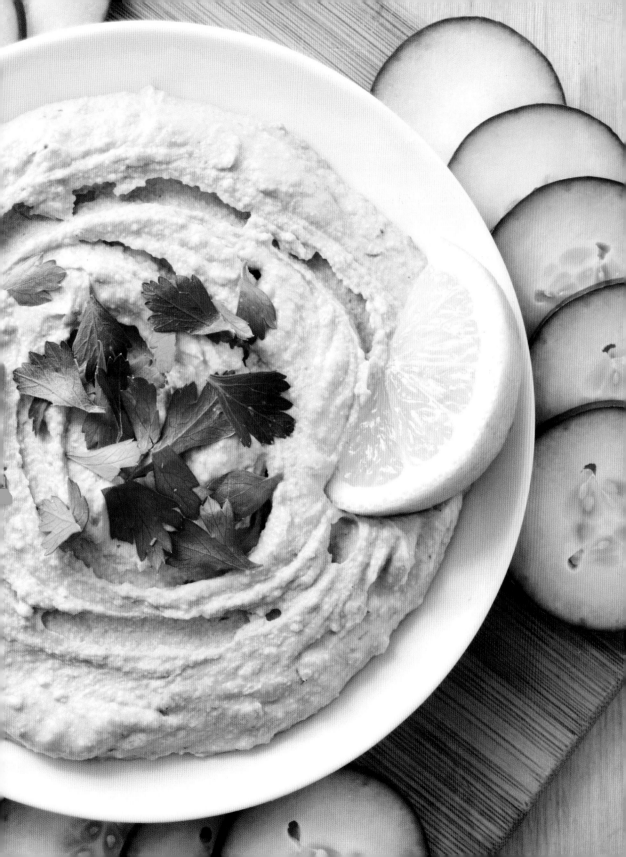

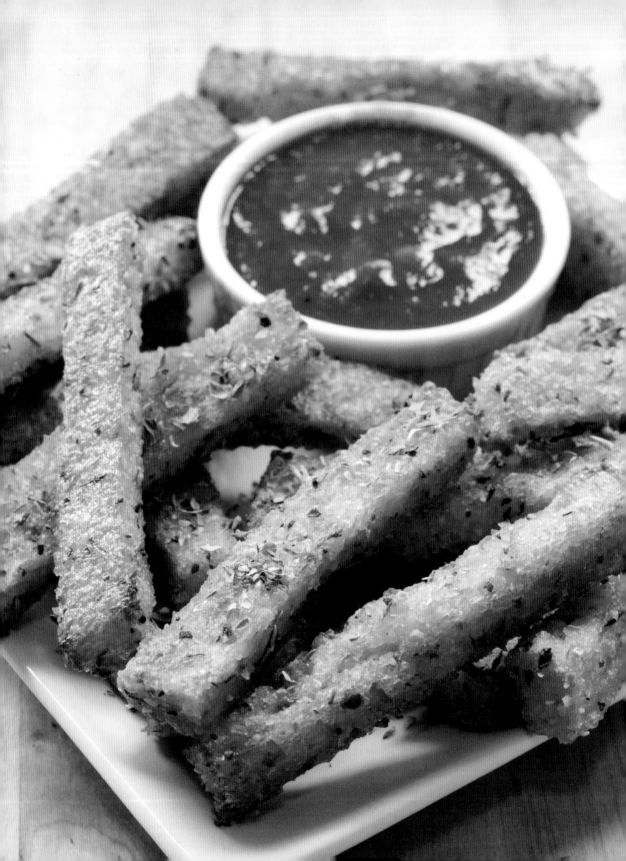

HERBED *polenta* FRIES

TOTAL TIME: 1 HOUR (PLUS TIME FOR CHILLING POLENTA) **ACTIVE TIME:** 30 MINUTES
MAKES: 6 SERVINGS

Fresh out of the oven, these fries are pure crispy-salty satisfaction. I'll often save time before serving them at dinner or a party by preparing the polenta the night before so it's ready to be quickly sliced, baked, and enjoyed warm.

FRIES
4 cups vegetable broth
1 cup coarse-ground cornmeal
3 tablespoons olive oil, divided
½ teaspoon garlic powder
½ teaspoon dried basil
½ teaspoon dried oregano
½ teaspoon dried rosemary
½ teaspoon dried thyme
Salt and black pepper, to taste

SERVING OPTIONS
Heated marinara sauce
Ketchup
Any other favorite dips

1. In a medium pot, bring the vegetable broth to a boil over high heat. Add the cornmeal, turn the heat down, and simmer for 20 minutes, stirring with a whisk or fork every 5 minutes.

2. Turn the heat off and stir in 1 tablespoon of the olive oil, plus the garlic powder, basil, oregano, rosemary, thyme, salt, and pepper.

3. Grease a 13-by-9-inch glass baking dish and pour the mixture into it. Place the polenta in the refrigerator to set for at least 1 hour (or overnight).

4. When the polenta is completely cool, remove it from the refrigerator. Preheat the oven to 450°F.

5. Gently flip the baking dish over onto a cutting board so the polenta easily slides out. Slice it into fries about ½ inch thick and 2 inches long.

6. Grease a baking sheet with 1 tablespoon of the olive oil. Spread the fries on the baking sheet and brush the tops with the remaining 1 tablespoon olive oil. Bake for 25 minutes. Remove from the oven and use a spatula to flip the fries. Return to the oven and bake for another 10–15 minutes, until the edges are crispy and golden.

7. Enjoy right away with marinara sauce, ketchup, or your favorite dip.

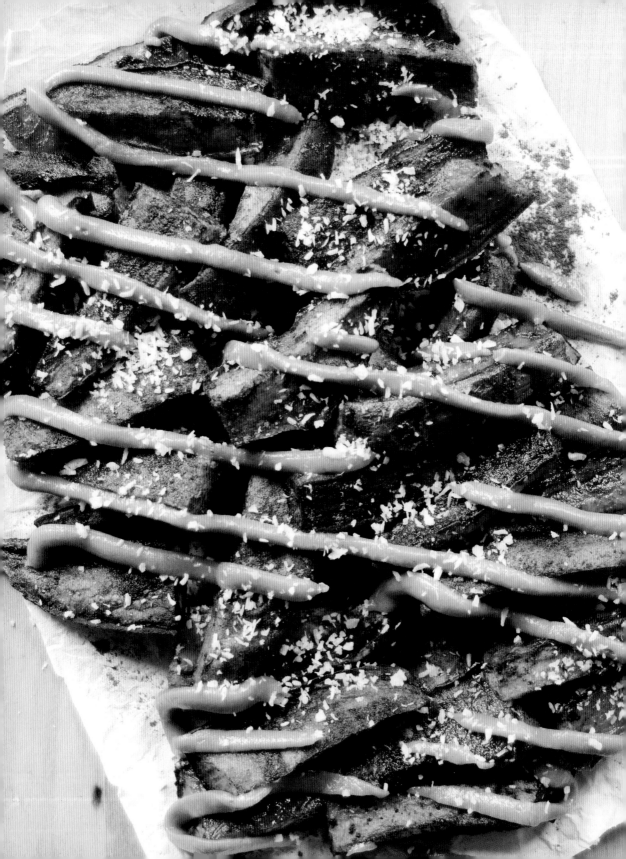

CINNAMON *sweet potato fries* WITH MAPLE PB SAUCE

TOTAL TIME: 45 MINUTES **ACTIVE TIME:** 15 MINUTES **MAKES:** 4 SERVINGS

Part side dish, part dessert, these fries answer the call of all cravings any time of the day.

FRIES
4 medium sweet potatoes
1 tablespoon coconut oil, melted
1 tablespoon coconut sugar
1 teaspoon ground cinnamon
⅛ teaspoon salt

SAUCE
2 tablespoons maple syrup
2 tablespoons peanut butter
2 tablespoons shredded coconut (optional)

1. Preheat the oven to 400°F.

2. Scrub the sweet potatoes and slice them into fries about ½ inch thick. Place them in a large bowl.

3. Toss the fries with the coconut oil, coconut sugar, cinnamon, and salt. Spread them out on a baking sheet.

4. Bake for 20 minutes. Remove from the oven and use a spatula to flip the fries. Return them to the oven for another 10 minutes.

5. While the fries bake, prepare the sauce by stirring the maple syrup and peanut butter together in a small cup. Serve the sauce on the side for dipping, or drizzle it on top of the fries. Sprinkle the shredded coconut over the fries, if desired.

COCONUT-CRUSTED *avocado* FRIES

⊕ **TOTAL TIME:** 35 MINUTES   **ACTIVE TIME:** 15 MINUTES   **MAKES:** 4 SERVINGS

Coconut and avocado are two of my all-time favorite ingredients. Together, they make crispy-on-the-outside, creamy-on-the-inside magic in these baked fries.

AVOCADO FRIES
2 ripe avocados

BATTER
¼ cup nondairy milk
1 tablespoon tamari
1 tablespoon olive oil
1 tablespoon maple syrup
1 cup shredded coconut
Salt and black pepper, to taste

SERVE WITH
Ketchup
½ batch Cashew Sour Cream
  (see page 226) or store-
  bought vegan sour cream

1. Preheat the oven to 400°F. Grease a baking sheet.

2. Peel and pit the avocados and cut them into ½-inch-thick slices.

3. To make the batter, in a small bowl, stir together the nondairy milk, tamari, olive oil, and maple syrup. Spread the shredded coconut out on a plate.

4. Dip the avocado slices into the batter, and then roll them in shredded coconut to coat. Place on the baking sheet and sprinkle with salt and pepper.

5. Bake for 15 minutes, then flip the fries and bake for another 5 minutes. Enjoy fresh out of the oven. Serve with ketchup and **Cashew Sour Cream**.

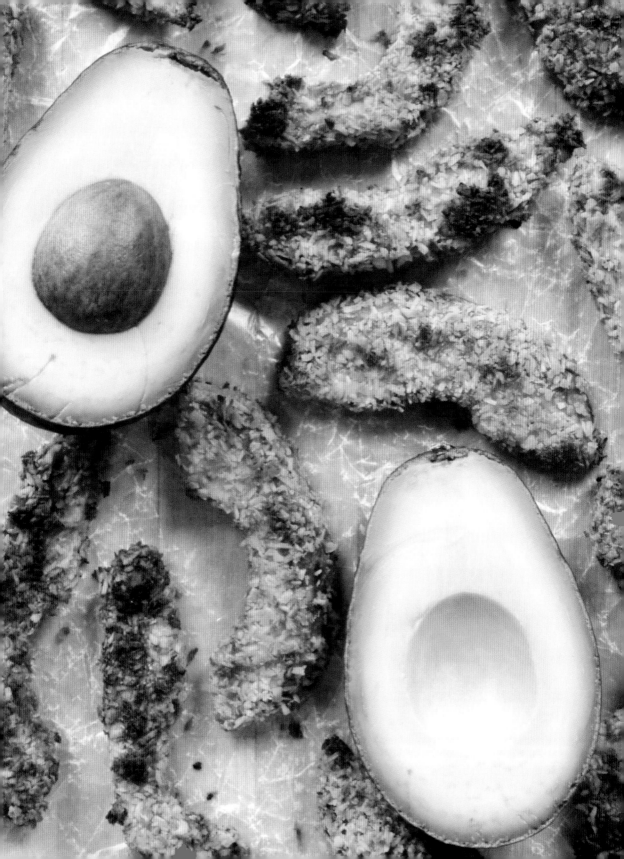

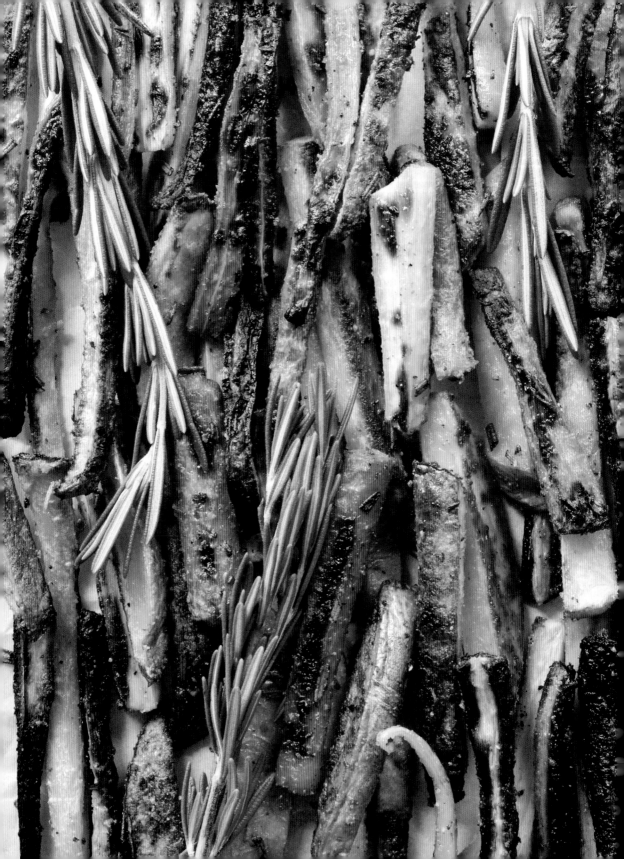

BAKED ROSEMARY
root vegetable FRIES

TOTAL TIME: 50 MINUTES   **ACTIVE TIME:** 10 MINUTES   **MAKES:** 4–6 SERVINGS

Spotting rainbow carrots at the farmer's market always makes my day. My favorite way to showcase their colorful glory is with these fries. This recipe is seriously simple, but the subtle hint of rosemary helps it pack an impressive punch.

6 large rainbow carrots
1 large parsnip
1 sweet potato
2 Yukon Gold potatoes
2 tablespoons olive oil
2 tablespoons chopped fresh
   rosemary
1 teaspoon garlic powder
1 teaspoon onion powder
Salt and black pepper, to taste

1. Preheat the oven to 400°F.

2. Peel the carrots, parsnip, sweet potato, and Yukon Gold potatoes, and slice them into fries about ½ inch thick and 2 inches long.

3. Place the veggie fries in a large bowl and toss with the olive oil, rosemary, garlic powder, onion powder, salt, and pepper.

4. Spread the fries out on a baking sheet. Bake for 20 minutes, flip, and bake for another 10–20 minutes (this will depend on the size of the fries), until crispy. Enjoy fresh out of the oven.

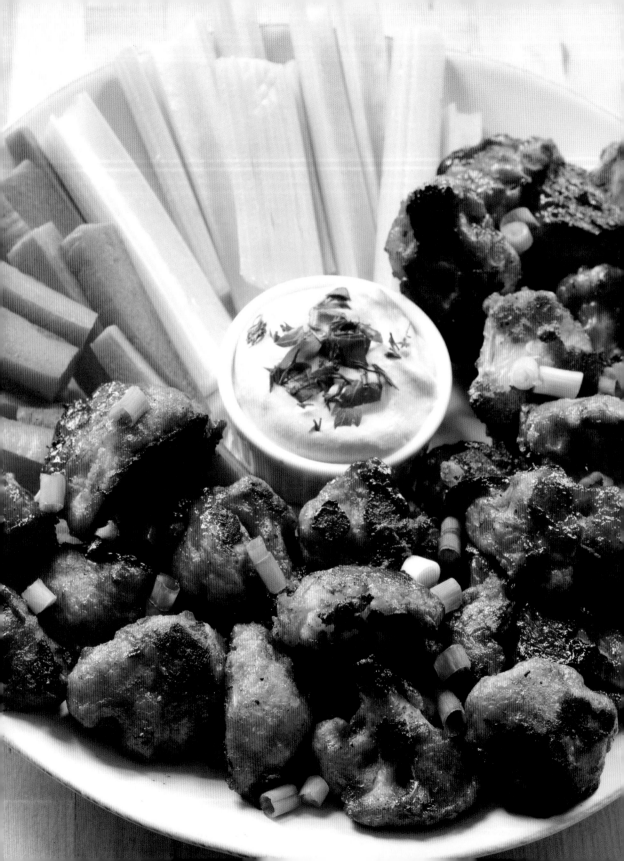

BBQ CAULIFLOWER
poppers

⊕ **TOTAL TIME:** 1 HOUR **ACTIVE TIME:** 15 MINUTES **MAKES:** 4–6 SERVINGS

When I first came up with this recipe, I made a batch for my mom to try. She liked it so much that she tried to trick me into making her another batch by remarking that something was off and we should keep testing the recipe. Good one, Mom. Double your batch and make BBQ Ranch Cauliflower Pizza (see page 170) the next day!

BATTER
½ cup spelt flour
¾ cup nondairy milk
1 tablespoon olive oil
½ teaspoon garlic powder
⅛ teaspoon salt

CAULIFLOWER
2 tablespoons olive oil
1 cauliflower crown, broken
   into florets
1 cup barbecue sauce

SERVE WITH
Green onions, sliced
1 batch Green Cashew Ranch
   Dressing (see page 234)
Celery sticks
Carrot sticks

1. Preheat the oven to 425°F.

2. Stir all the batter ingredients together in a small bowl.

3. Grease a baking sheet with the olive oil. Dip the cauliflower florets into the batter and place them on the baking sheet.

4. Bake for 15 minutes, then flip the cauliflower with a spatula and bake for 5 more minutes.

5. Remove the baking sheet from the oven. Carefully transfer the cauliflower to a large bowl. Add the barbecue sauce and stir until all the pieces are coated.

6. Spread the cauliflower out on the baking sheet. Bake for another 15 minutes, then flip the cauliflower and bake for another 10 minutes, until crispy.

7. Let the cauliflower cool for 5 minutes, then garnish with the green onions and serve with the Green Cashew Ranch Dressing, celery sticks, and carrot sticks.

LOADED *ranch* POTATO SALAD

⊕ **TOTAL TIME:** 30 MINUTES   **ACTIVE TIME:** 10 MINUTES   **MAKES:** 6 SERVINGS

This is no boring side dish. Perfect for picnics and summer barbecues, this potato salad goes great with grilled veggies, burgers, and sandwiches.

2 pounds red potatoes

1 batch Tempeh Bacon (see page 231), sliced into small pieces

4 celery stalks, diced

2 green onions, sliced

2 tablespoons chopped fresh parsley

2 tablespoons chopped fresh dill

½ batch Green Cashew Ranch Dressing (see page 234)

Salt and black pepper, to taste

1. Bring a large pot of water to a boil over high heat. If the potatoes are on the large side, slice them in half. Put the potatoes in the pot and boil until tender, 15–20 minutes.

2. Drain the potatoes and rinse with cold water until they're cool. Slice them into bite-size pieces and transfer them to a large bowl.

3. Add the Tempeh Bacon, celery, green onions, parsley, dill, Green Cashew Ranch Dressing, salt, and pepper to the bowl and stir. Serve fresh or store in the refrigerator for later.

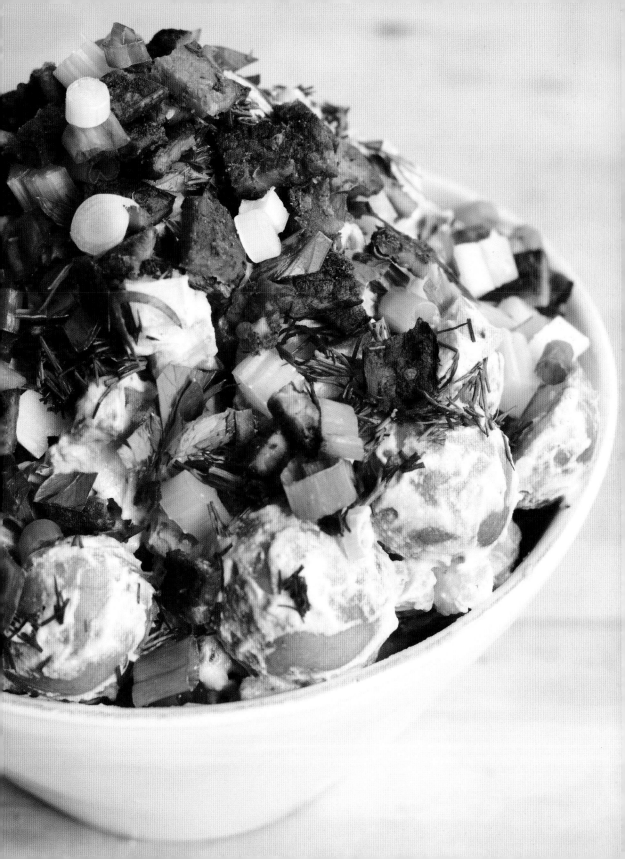

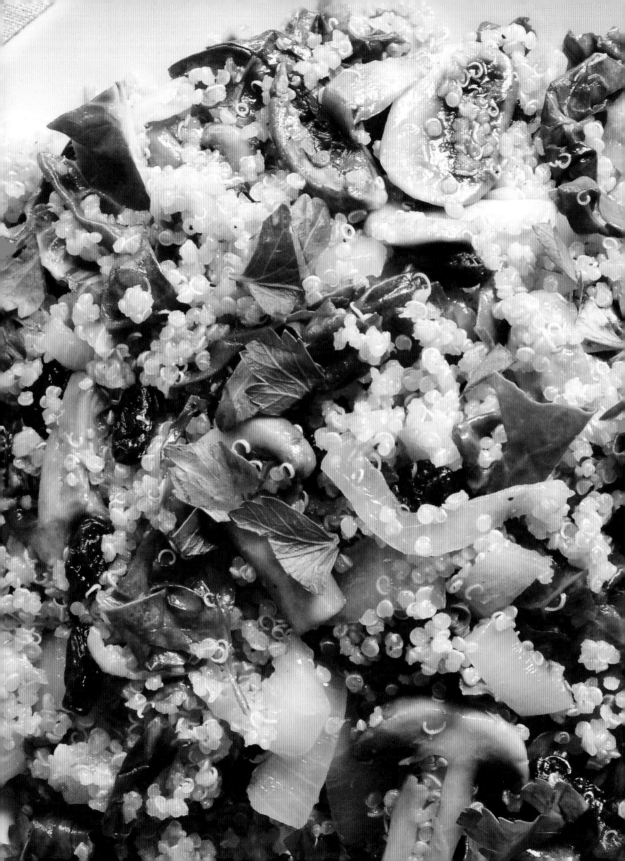

mushroom QUINOA

⊕ **TOTAL TIME:** 20 MINUTES **MAKES:** 4 SERVINGS

Quinoa is a great way to get in extra protein and fiber, and this side dish will round out just about any meal. I like to serve this yummy and filling dish alongside Sweet & Savory Sweet Potato Soup (see page 91) and Whole Roasted Tahini Cauliflower (see page 153).

2 tablespoons olive oil, divided
1 medium onion, sliced
2 cloves garlic, minced
2 cups sliced button or cremini mushrooms
2 cups packed shredded Swiss chard
⅓ cup raisins
1 batch Quinoa (see page 228)
Salt and black pepper, to taste
2 tablespoons chopped fresh parsley

1. In a medium pan, heat 1 tablespoon of the olive oil over medium-high heat. Add the onion and garlic and sauté for 3 minutes.

2. Turn the heat down to medium and add the mushrooms. Sauté for 5–7 minutes, until the mushrooms are lightly browned. Add the chard and raisins and sauté until the chard wilts, 2–3 minutes.

3. Stir in the Quinoa, remaining 1 tablespoon olive oil, salt, and pepper. Cook until everything is warm, then transfer to plates and top with the parsley.

CREAMY BAKED KALE
& *artichoke* DIP

TOTAL TIME: 45 MINUTES **ACTIVE TIME:** 25 MINUTES **MAKES:** 12 SERVINGS

While I was in the recipe-testing stage of writing this book, my friend Talia tried this recipe for her annual Friendsgiving party (a pre–Thanksgiving Day gathering of friends). I hung out by the snack table to listen to people's reactions (and of course to eat all the snacks) and was thrilled to learn that no one even guessed it was dairy-free.

CREAM

1 (13½-ounce) can full-fat coconut milk
1½ cups cooked white beans (or one 15-ounce can, rinsed and drained)
½ cup nutritional yeast
Juice of 1 lemon

SAUTÉED KALE

1 tablespoon olive oil
1 medium onion, diced
3 cloves garlic, minced
6 cups shredded kale

EVERYTHING ELSE

3 cups chopped artichoke hearts (or two 15-ounce cans, drained and chopped)
Salt and black pepper, to taste

SERVING OPTIONS

Crackers
Chips
Toast

1. Preheat the oven to 400°F.

2. To prepare the cream, combine all the ingredients in a blender and blend until smooth. Set aside.

3. To prepare the sautéed kale, heat the olive oil over medium-high heat in a cast iron skillet.* Add the onion and garlic and sauté for 5 minutes. Turn the heat off, add the kale, and cook for 1–2 minutes, until the kale wilts.

4. Pour the cream mixture into the skillet. Add the artichoke hearts, salt, and pepper, and stir until thoroughly mixed.

5. Place the skillet in the oven and bake for 20 minutes, until bubbly. Remove from the oven and enjoy warm with crackers, chips, or toast.

NOTE: *Don't have a cast iron skillet? Use a regular pan, then transfer the mixture to a baking dish to bake.*

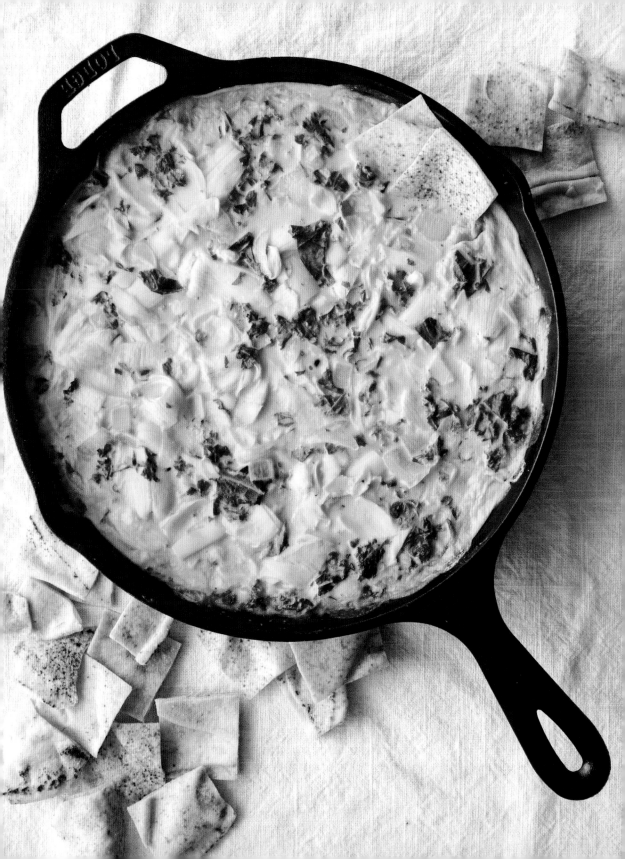

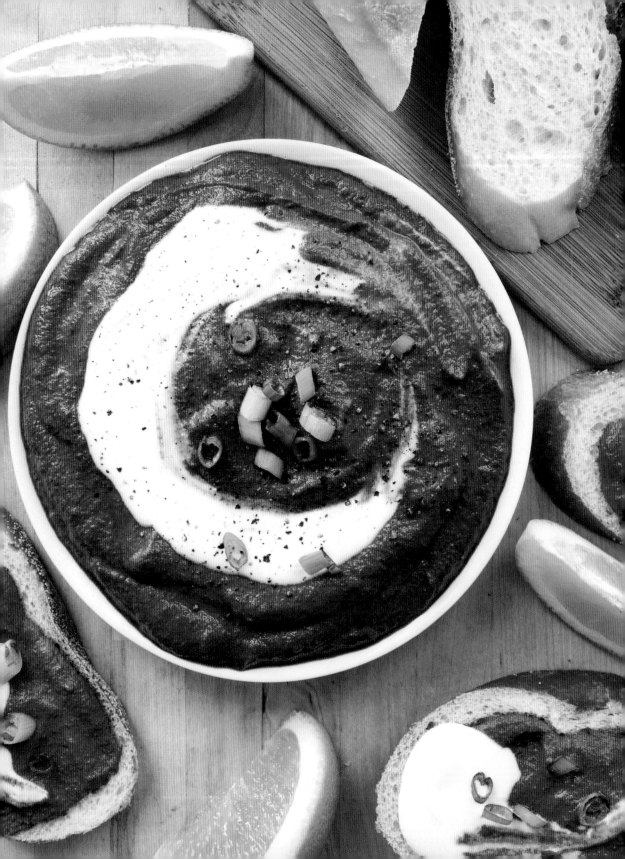

balsamic BEET SPREAD

⊕ **TOTAL TIME:** 50 MINUTES **ACTIVE TIME:** 10 MINUTES **MAKES:** 8–10 SERVINGS

I just can't get enough of the color of this pretty dip. This recipe makes a fun alternative to hummus and is great as a spread for crackers or a dip for fresh veggies.

BEET SPREAD

3 medium beets, peeled and cut into 1-inch pieces (about 2 cups)

2 tablespoons olive oil, divided

1½ cups cooked chickpeas (or one 15-ounce can, rinsed and drained)

Juice of ½ orange

¼ cup tahini

2 tablespoons balsamic vinegar

2 tablespoons maple syrup (or more for a sweeter dip)

1 clove garlic, crushed

Salt and black pepper, to taste

TOPPINGS

½ batch Cashew Sour Cream (see page 226) or store-bought vegan sour cream

2 tablespoons chopped green onions

1. Preheat the oven to 400°F. In a medium bowl, toss the beets with 1 tablespoon of the olive oil, then spread them out on a baking sheet. Bake for 40 minutes, until tender when poked with a fork.

2. When the beets are cool enough to handle, transfer them to a blender and add the remaining 1 tablespoon olive oil, chickpeas, orange juice, tahini, balsamic vinegar, maple syrup, garlic, salt, and pepper. Blend until smooth.

3. Transfer the mixture to a serving dish. Top with the Cashew Sour Cream and green onions.

STRAWBERRY *mango* SALSA

TOTAL TIME: 10 MINUTES   **MAKES:** 6–8 SERVINGS

Hello, summer! Sweet and spicy, this salsa tastes like sunshine on a chip. I think it's best enjoyed with a margarita in one hand.

SALSA
2 cups diced mango (about 2 fruits)
2 cups diced strawberries
2 tablespoons diced red onion
2 tablespoons chopped fresh cilantro
½–1 jalapeño pepper, seeded and minced
Juice of 1 lime
1 tablespoon maple syrup
Dash of salt

SERVE WITH
Tortilla chips

1. Toss all the salsa ingredients together in a bowl. Serve fresh with the tortilla chips.

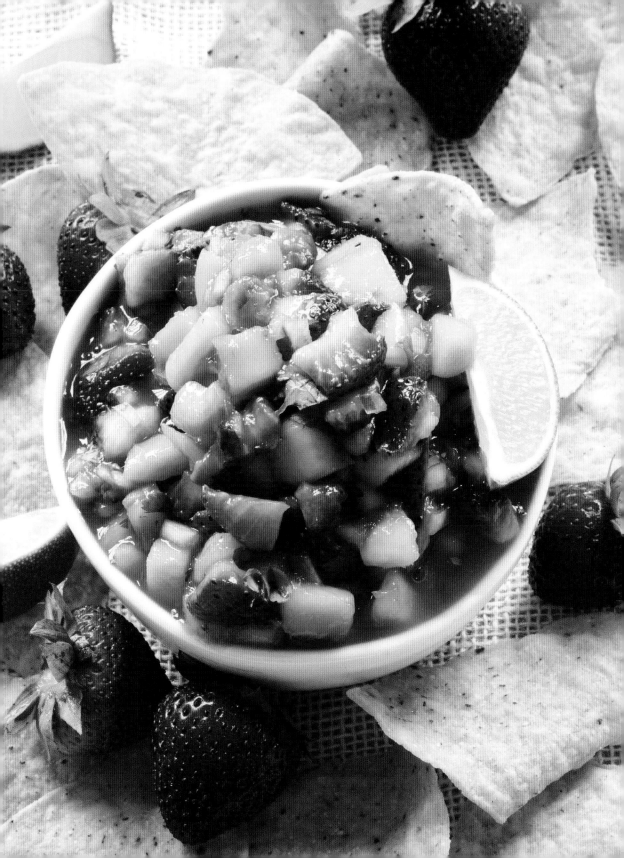

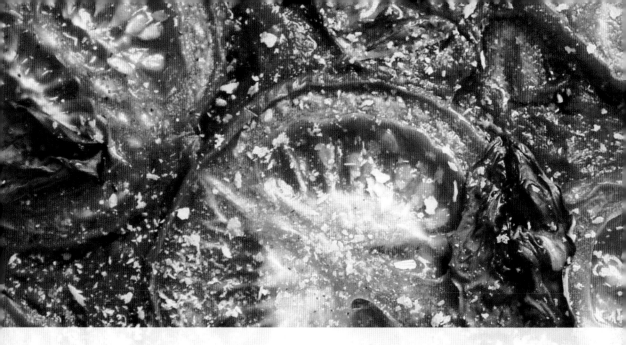

entrées

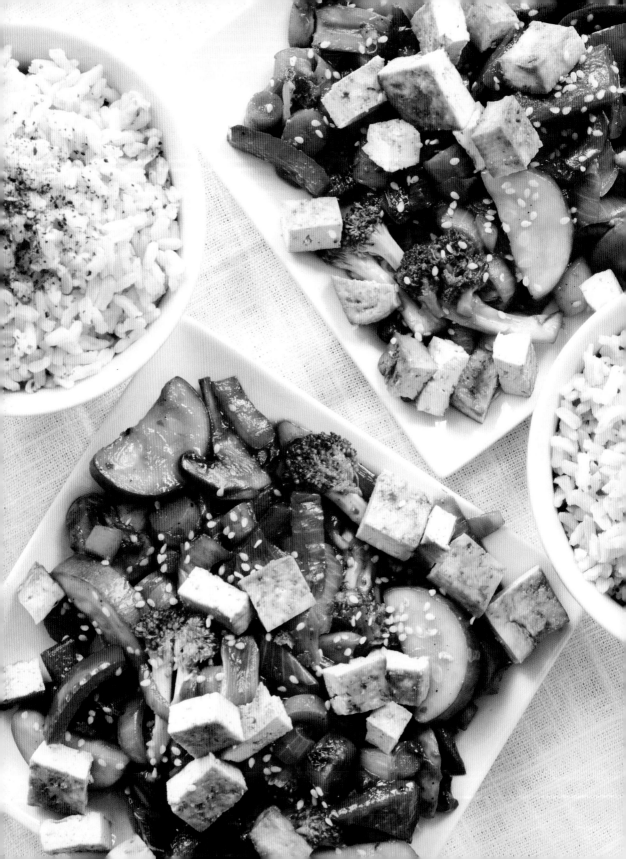

VEGETABLE *teriyaki* STIR-FRY

⊕ **TOTAL TIME:** 20 MINUTES **MAKES:** 4 SERVINGS

If you can chop and stir, you can make a delicious, better-than-takeout stir-fry. Use this recipe as a starting point and get creative with whatever veggies are in season. You can't go wrong!

STIR-FRY
1 tablespoon coconut oil
1 medium onion, sliced
2 cloves garlic, minced
1 broccoli crown, broken into florets (about 2 cups)
1 red bell pepper, chopped
1 zucchini, sliced
2 cups sliced button or cremini mushrooms
1 cup chopped carrot
1 batch Teriyaki Sauce (see page 237)

SERVE WITH
1 batch Baked Tofu (see page 233)
1 batch Brown Rice (see page 228)
Sesame seeds

1. In a large pan or wok, heat the coconut oil over medium-high heat. Add the onion and garlic and sauté for 3 minutes.

2. Turn the heat down to medium and add the broccoli, bell pepper, zucchini, mushrooms, and carrot. Sauté for about 10 minutes, until everything is tender. Stir in the **Teriyaki Sauce** and heat until warm.

3. Transfer to plates, serve with the **Baked Tofu** and **Brown Rice**, and sprinkle with the sesame seeds.

STIR-FRY IT . . . EVERY WEEKNIGHT!

Teriyaki sauce may be the most traditional stir-fry flavor, but I love getting wild with different sauces. Make a totally different stir-fry every weeknight by swapping in one of the sauces below and serving it over quinoa, lentils, or soba or brown rice noodles.

Peanut Sauce (see page 236)
Cashew Cheese Sauce (see page 239)

Green Tahini Sauce (see page 238)
Cauliflower Alfredo Sauce (see page 239)

CREAMY *coconut polenta* WITH BALSAMIC MUSHROOMS & CHICKPEAS

TOTAL TIME: 45 MINUTES **MAKES:** 4 SERVINGS

My husband and I got married during the summer, in a beautifully renovated barn in upstate New York. We strung twinkle lights across the ceiling, lined the farm-style tables with lace, and covered the tables with plants and flowers. We wanted the menu to match the rustic atmosphere, so we served grilled summer vegetables over creamy polenta (plus a three-tiered vegan double-chocolate cake). Since then, polenta has been a staple in our house, especially this version that's made extra thick and creamy with the help of coconut milk.

POLENTA BASE
1 cup medium-ground cornmeal
1 (13½-ounce can) full-fat coconut milk
4 cups vegetable broth

MUSHROOM TOPPING
1 tablespoon coconut oil
1 medium onion, sliced
2 cloves garlic, minced
4 cups button or cremini mushrooms, sliced in half
3 tablespoons balsamic vinegar
1 tablespoon maple syrup
1 tablespoon water
1½ cups cooked chickpeas (or one 15-ounce can, rinsed and drained)
3 cups packed baby spinach
Salt and black pepper, to taste

1. To prepare the polenta, combine the cornmeal, coconut milk, and vegetable broth in a medium saucepan. Bring to a boil over medium-high heat, then reduce the heat and simmer for 30 minutes, stirring every 5 minutes. Turn the heat off and let the polenta sit for 5 minutes before serving.

2. While the polenta cooks, prepare the mushroom topping. Heat the coconut oil in a pan over medium-high heat. Add the onion and garlic and sauté for 5 minutes.

3. Add the mushrooms, balsamic vinegar, maple syrup, and water. Cook for about 8 minutes, stirring occasionally, until the mushrooms are tender.

4. Add the chickpeas and cook for 1–2 minutes, until heated. Turn the heat off and stir in the spinach until it wilts, about 2 minutes.

5. To serve, transfer the polenta to a large bowl and top with the mushroom mixture. Season with salt and pepper.

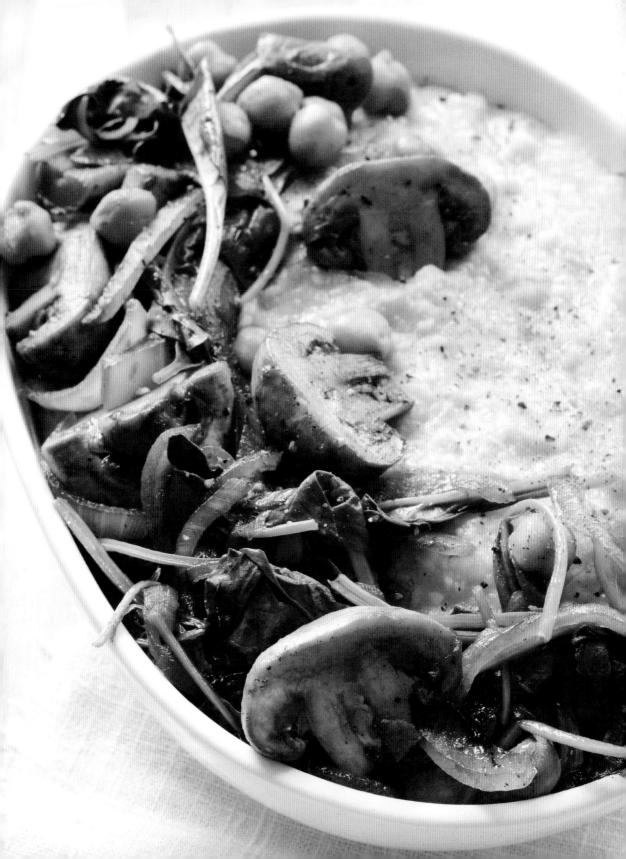

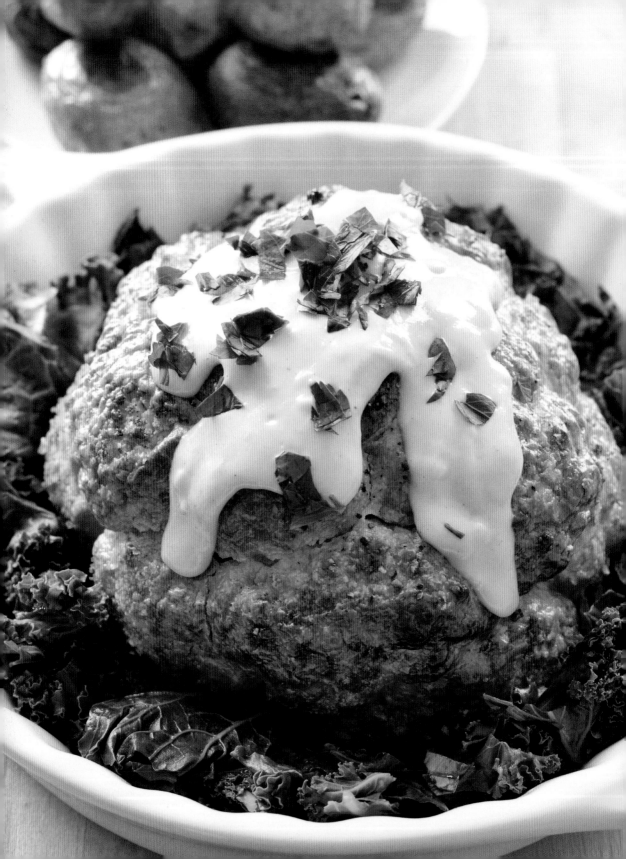

WHOLE ROASTED *tahini* CAULIFLOWER

TOTAL TIME: 1 HOUR 15 MINUTES   **ACTIVE TIME:** 15 MINUTES   **MAKES:** 4 SERVINGS

The first time I made this recipe I had originally set out to make roasted tahini cauliflower bites, but I ended up feeling a little lazy so I decided to see what would happen if I skipped a step and didn't chop the cauliflower. The result was the most heavenly, melt-in-your-mouth dish ever—my laziness totally paid off! For a complete meal, I like to serve it with Mushroom Quinoa (see page 139).

CAULIFLOWER BASE
1 medium cauliflower crown

TAHINI SAUCE
¼ cup tahini
Juice of 1 lemon
3 tablespoons olive oil
1 tablespoon water
2 teaspoons tamari
2 cloves garlic, minced

TOPPINGS
Salt and black pepper, to taste
2 tablespoons chopped
   fresh parsley

1. Preheat the oven to 400°F. Line a baking sheet with aluminum foil.

2. Rinse the cauliflower, trim off the leaves, and cut the stem so that the cauliflower will sit upright on the baking sheet and the sauce will coat the top.

3. In a small bowl, stir all the tahini sauce ingredients together. Using a pastry brush, coat the cauliflower with the tahini sauce, using about half of the sauce and reserving the rest for later. Sprinkle salt and pepper over the cauliflower.

4. Roast the cauliflower for 55–60 minutes, until the outside is crispy and brown. Warm the remaining sauce in a small saucepan over low heat, then drizzle it over the cauliflower. Sprinkle the parsley on top. Use a knife to slice the cauliflower and serve warm.

EGGPLANT & ZUCCHINI *no-noodle* LASAGNA

⊕ **TOTAL TIME:** 1 HOUR 30 MINUTES **ACTIVE TIME:** 30 MINUTES **MAKES:** 4–6 SERVINGS

One of my mom's favorite stories is about my childhood fascination with lasagna. She would make multiple, gigantic lasagnas whenever our cousins came to visit, and I would hover around her in the kitchen, making her repeat the order of the layers until I could recite it by memory. Well, apparently my fascination still holds up because this recipe is all about the layers, baby!

3 tablespoons olive oil, divided
1 medium eggplant
3 medium zucchini
1 (24-ounce) jar marinara sauce
1 batch Cashew Cheese
   Sauce (see page 239)
2 medium tomatoes, sliced
1 handful fresh basil
1 tablespoon nutritional yeast
Salt and black pepper, to taste

1. Preheat the oven to 400°F. Lightly coat two baking sheets with 1 tablespoon of the olive oil.

2. To prepare the eggplant and zucchini "noodles," cut the tops and bottoms off the eggplant and zucchini. Slice them lengthwise into strips about ½ inch thick. Place them on the baking sheets and brush with 1 tablespoon of the olive oil.

3. Bake for 20 minutes, flipping halfway through the cooking time. Remove and set aside.

4. Turn the oven down to 375°F. Assemble the lasagna by spreading a thin layer of the marinara sauce across the bottom of an 11-by-7-inch glass baking dish. Place a layer of zucchini "noodles" on top. Spread a thin layer of the **Cashew Cheese Sauce** over the zucchini, followed by another thin layer of marinara sauce. Repeat the process, using the eggplant "noodles." Continue repeating until all the "noodles" are used (about 4 layers total).

5. Spread a thin layer of marinara sauce on top, and top with the tomatoes and basil. Drizzle with the remaining 1 tablespoon of olive oil, and sprinkle nutritional yeast, salt, and pepper on top.

6. Cover and bake for 20 minutes, until the lasagna begins to bubble. Uncover and bake for 15–20 more minutes, until the tomatoes are crispy. Let the dish sit for 10 minutes before serving. Enjoy warm.

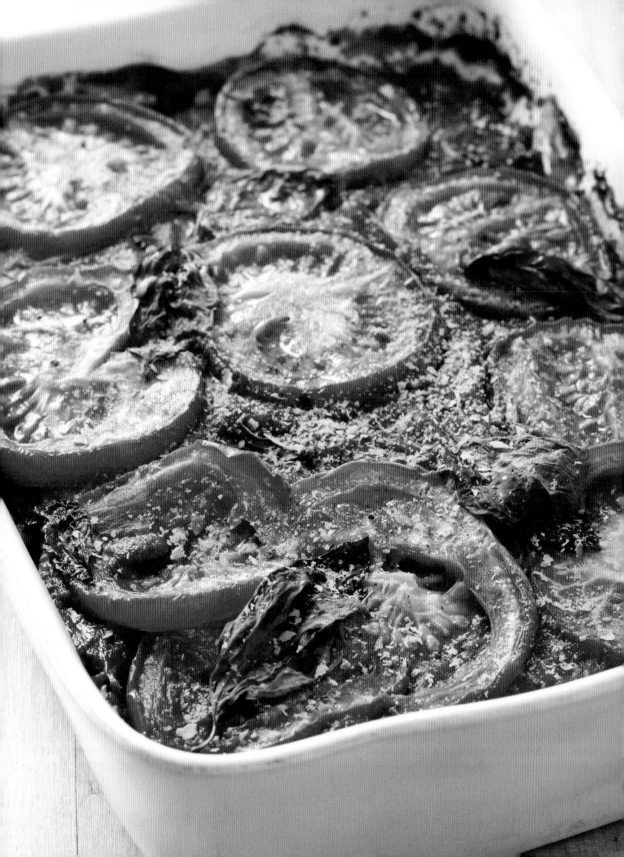

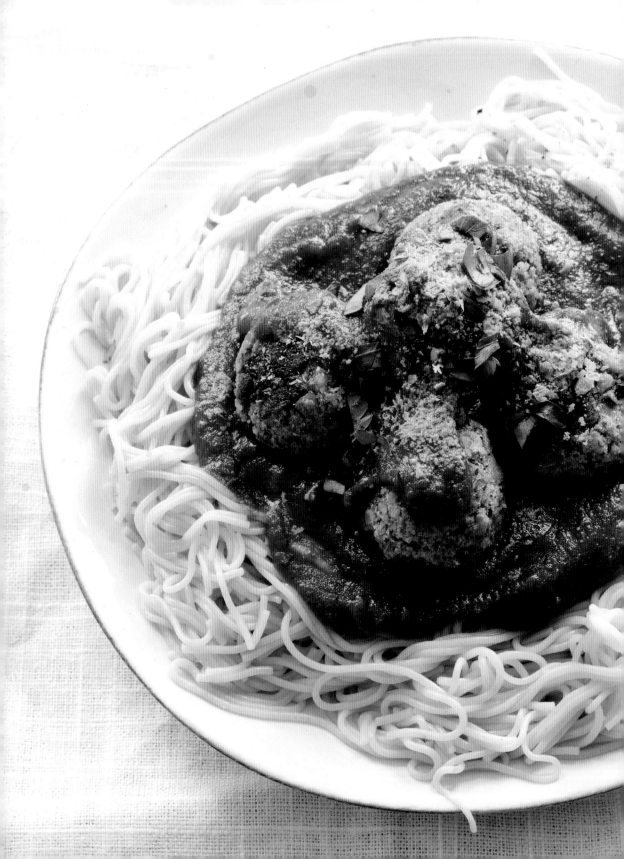

SPAGHETTI & *tempeh-mushroom* MEATBALLS

TOTAL TIME: 40 MINUTES **ACTIVE TIME:** 20 MINUTES
MAKES: 4 SERVINGS (ABOUT 20 MEATBALLS)

Crispy on the outside and soft on the inside, these "meatballs" are a flavor and texture dream. Whip up an easy weeknight dinner by serving them over your favorite pasta and sauce. Use the leftovers to make Meatball & Garlicky Greens Subs *(see page 117) the next day.*

MEATBALLS
3 tablespoons olive oil, divided
1 tablespoon ground flaxseed
3 tablespoons warm water
1 small onion, diced
2 cloves garlic, minced
2 cups diced button or
     cremini mushrooms
1 (8-ounce) package tempeh,
     crumbled
1 tablespoon tamari
1 teaspoon dried oregano
1 teaspoon dried basil
½ cup breadcrumbs, plus
     extra if needed
Salt and black pepper, to taste

BASES AND TOPPINGS
4 servings of spaghetti,
     uncooked
4 servings of your favorite
     sauce
Nutritional yeast
Chopped fresh parsley

1. Preheat the oven to 400°F. Grease a baking sheet with 1 tablespoon of the olive oil.

2. Prepare a flax "egg" by stirring the ground flaxseed and warm water together in a small bowl. Let the mixture sit for at least 10 minutes before using.

3. Heat 1 tablespoon of the olive oil in a pan over medium-high heat. Add the onion, garlic, and mushrooms, and sauté for 5 minutes.

4. Transfer the mushroom mixture to a blender or food processor. Add the flax "egg," tempeh, tamari, oregano, and basil, and pulse until a moldable texture is formed.

5. Transfer the mixture to a large bowl. Stir in the breadcrumbs, adding enough so that the dough can be easily rolled into balls. Add salt and pepper. Wet your hands and roll the mixture into balls, using 1 heaping tablespoon per ball. Place the balls on the baking sheet and brush the tops with the remaining 1 tablespoon olive oil.

6. Bake for 20 minutes, using a spatula to flip the meatballs halfway through.

7. While the meatballs bake, prepare the pasta according to the instructions on the package. Heat the sauce in a small saucepan.

8. Transfer the pasta to individual bowls, then top each bowl with sauce. Serve the meatballs over everything and sprinkle with the nutritional yeast and parsley.

SWEET POTATO & *greens* MAC 'N' CHEESE

TOTAL TIME: 1 HOUR 10 MINUTES   **ACTIVE TIME:** 10 MINUTES   **MAKES:** 6 SERVINGS

This dish is the number-one most popular on The Colorful Kitchen *blog—and one of my personal favorites, too. Many readers have mentioned that it's a hit with friends and family who tend to be skeptical of anything labeled "vegan." I like to double or triple the sauce recipe and freeze individual portions for mac 'n' cheese emergencies.*

1 large sweet potato
6 servings of your favorite pasta, uncooked (I like gluten-free brown rice "elbows")
1 cup nondairy milk
2 cloves garlic, crushed
1 tablespoon Dijon mustard
¼ cup nutritional yeast
2 tablespoons tamari
1 tablespoon olive oil
Salt and black pepper, to taste
2 cups packed greens of your choice

1. Preheat the oven to 400°F. Use a knife to poke holes in the sweet potato, and place it on a baking sheet. Bake for 45–60 minutes, until the sweet potato is tender.

2. While the sweet potato bakes, prepare the pasta according to the instructions on the package.

3. Remove the sweet potato from the oven. When it's cool enough to handle, peel away the skin, scoop out the flesh, and put it in a blender.

4. Add the nondairy milk, garlic, mustard, nutritional yeast, tamari, olive oil, salt, and pepper to the blender, and blend until smooth.

5. In a large pot over medium heat, heat the greens with 1 tablespoon of water until they wilt, 2–3 minutes. Stir in the sweet potato sauce and pasta, and heat until warm, 4–5 minutes. Spoon into bowls and serve.

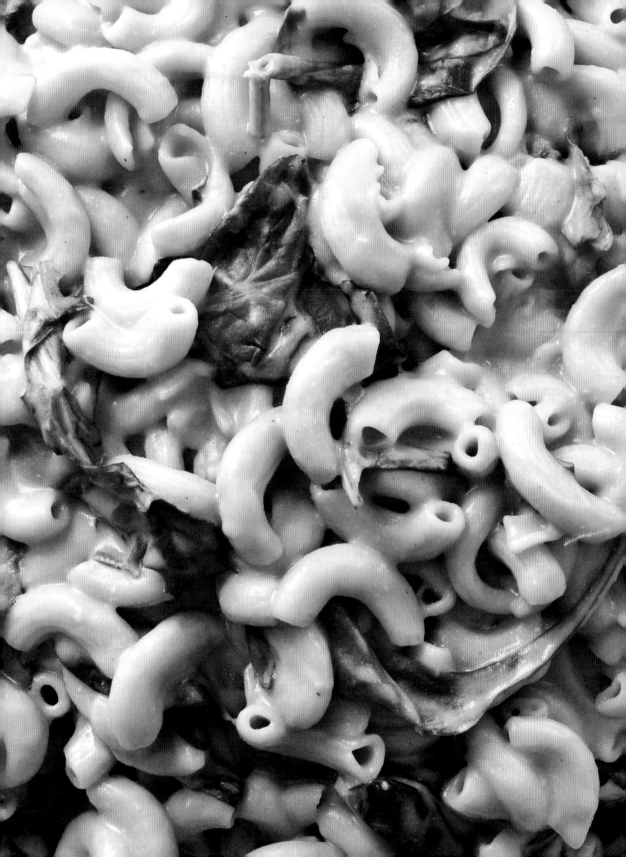

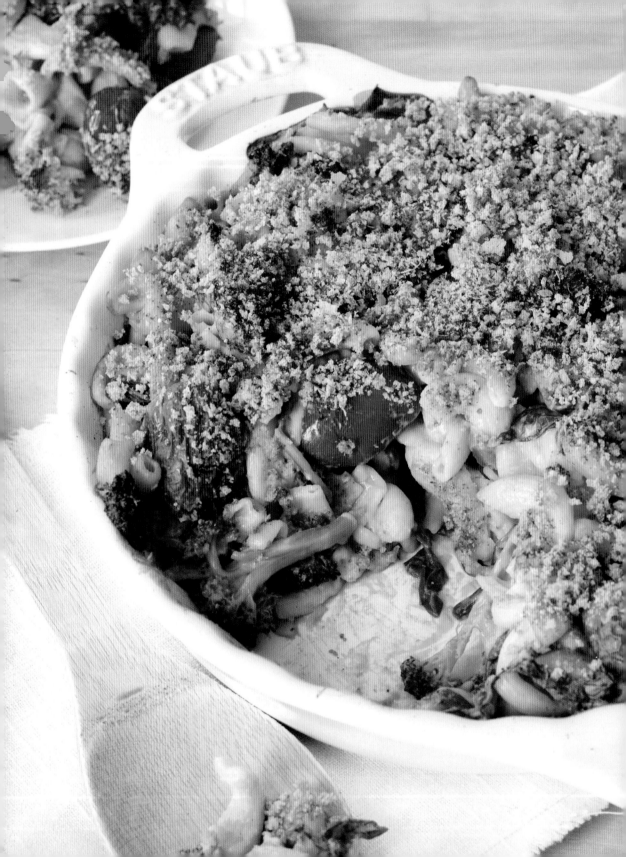

VEGGIE MAC *casserole*

⊕ **TOTAL TIME:** 50 MINUTES **ACTIVE TIME:** 10 MINUTES **MAKES:** 6 SERVINGS

If you're the kind of person who can eat mac 'n' cheese every night, try doubling the Sweet Potato & Greens Mac 'n' Cheese recipe and throwing this easy casserole together the next day.

2 tablespoons olive oil, divided
1 red bell pepper, chopped
1 cup cherry tomatoes
1 broccoli crown, broken into
　florets (about 2 cups)
1 batch Sweet Potato &
　Greens Mac 'n' Cheese
　(see page 158), leftover or
　freshly made
½ cup breadcrumbs
1 tablespoon nutritional yeast
½ teaspoon paprika
Salt and black pepper, to taste

1. Preheat the oven to 425°F. Grease a 9-by-9-inch casserole dish with 1 tablespoon of the olive oil.

2. In a bowl, toss the bell pepper, cherry tomatoes, and broccoli with the remaining 1 tablespoon olive oil. Spread the vegetables out on a baking sheet. Bake for 20 minutes, flipping halfway through the baking time.

3. Remove the vegetables from the oven, and turn the heat down to 375°F.

4. In a large bowl, stir the roasted vegetables and the **Sweet Potato & Greens Mac 'n' Cheese** together. Transfer to the casserole dish and spread out evenly.

5. Sprinkle the breadcrumbs, nutritional yeast, paprika, salt, and pepper on top. Bake in the oven for 20–25 minutes, until the top is crispy. Enjoy fresh out of the oven or freeze for later.

SWEET POTATO & *spinach* GNOCCHI

TOTAL TIME: 1 HOUR 30 MINUTES **ACTIVE TIME:** 30 MINUTES **MAKES:** 4–6 SERVINGS

These gnocchi require more hands-on work than most of the recipes in this book, but for me, enjoying fresh, homemade gnocchi, especially on Sunday nights with the whole family, is totally worth it. All fried up, they're crispy on the outside and pillowy on the inside—a texture that simply cannot be rivaled by frozen versions.

GNOCCHI
3 medium sweet potatoes
3 cups packed spinach
⅛ teaspoon salt
2 cups spelt flour, plus extra
  for sprinkling
1–3 tablespoons olive oil

GARLIC & CHERRY TOMATO SAUCE
1 tablespoon olive oil
2 cloves garlic, minced
1 cup cherry tomatoes, sliced
  in half
1 bunch kale, chopped
Salt and black pepper, to taste

1. To roast the sweet potatoes, preheat the oven to 400°F. Line a baking sheet with parchment paper. Use a knife to poke holes in the sweet potatoes, and place them on the baking sheet. Bake for 45–60 minutes, until tender. Remove the sweet potatoes from the oven, and let them sit until they are cool enough to handle. Use a spoon to scoop the flesh into a large bowl.

2. Put the spinach in a large pot and add a few tablespoons of water. Heat the pot over medium-high heat, and stir until the spinach wilts, about 2 minutes. Transfer the spinach to a cutting board and rinse out the pot, saving it to boil the gnocchi in later.

3. When the spinach is cool enough to handle, finely chop it. Add it to the bowl with the sweet potato. Add the ⅛ teaspoon salt. Stir in the flour ½ cup at a time, until a dry but workable dough is formed. Divide into 4 balls.

4. Sprinkle more flour on a clean surface. Using your hands, roll each ball of dough out into a log about ½ inch thick. Use a knife to slice each log into 1-inch pieces.

5. Fill the large pot with water, and bring it to a boil over high heat. Gently lower the gnocchi into the water (you'll want to do this in two or three batches) and boil until they float to the top, about 4 minutes. With a slotted spoon, scoop the floating gnocchi out and place on a cooling rack to dry.

6. In a large pan, heat 1 tablespoon of the olive oil over medium heat. Add the gnocchi and fry for 4–5 minutes on each side, until browned. Repeat, adding more olive oil, until all the gnocchi are fried. Set aside.

7. Use the same pan to make the garlic & cherry tomato sauce. Heat the 1 tablespoon olive oil. Add the garlic and cook for 1 minute. Add the cherry tomatoes and cook for 1 more minute. Add the kale and cook for 1–2 minutes, until the kale wilts.

8. Turn the heat off and stir in the gnocchi. Sprinkle with salt and pepper and serve right away.

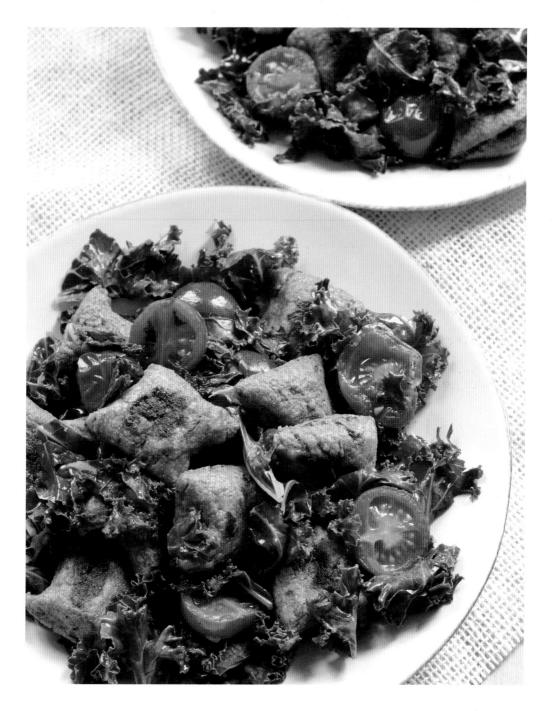

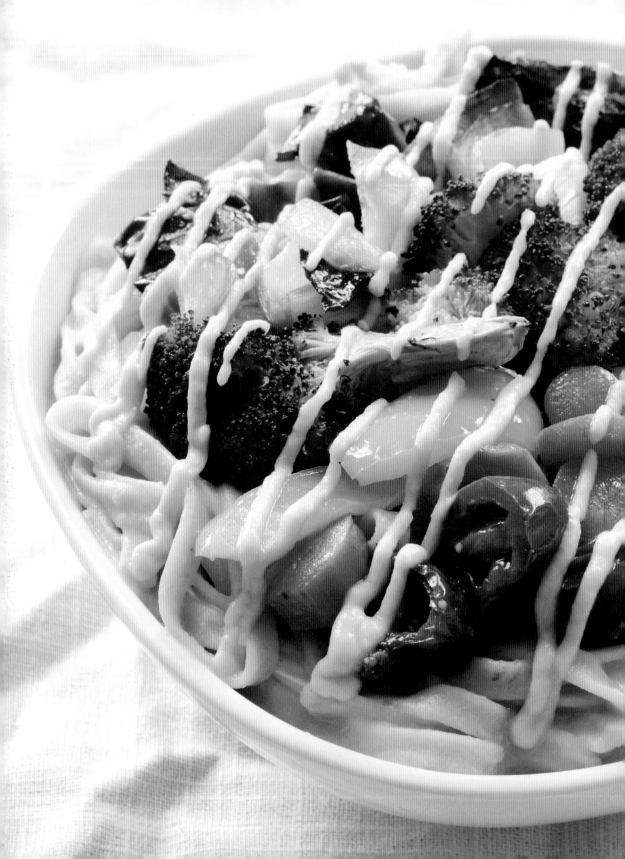

RAINBOW *cauliflower* ALFREDO PASTA

⊕ **TOTAL TIME:** 35 MINUTES   **ACTIVE TIME:** 20 MINUTES   **MAKES:** 4 SERVINGS

I can vividly remember the stomachaches I used to get after eating pasta with Alfredo sauce. I loved it too much to give it up, but boy did I pay the price. This lightened-up cauliflower-based version is rich, buttery, and creamy, without any of the heaviness. Both my heart and stomach stay happy post-meal. If you double your batch of sauce and roasted vegetables, you can make Chickpea Crust Rainbow Alfredo Pizza (see page 166) the next day.

RAINBOW ROASTED VEGETABLES

1 cup cherry tomatoes, sliced in half
1 cup chopped carrot
1 yellow bell pepper, chopped
1 cup broccoli florets
1 medium red onion, sliced
1 cup sliced purple cabbage
2 tablespoons olive oil
Salt and black pepper, to taste

ALFREDO PASTA

4 servings of your favorite pasta, uncooked
1 batch Cauliflower Alfredo Sauce (see page 239)

1. To prepare the rainbow roasted vegetables, preheat the oven to 400°F. Combine the cherry tomatoes, carrot, bell pepper, broccoli, onion, and cabbage in a large bowl. Add the olive oil, salt, and pepper and toss to combine. Spread the vegetables out on a baking sheet. Bake for 30–35 minutes, flipping the vegetables halfway through the baking time.

2. While the vegetables cook, make the Alfredo pasta. Prepare the pasta according to the instructions on the package.

3. Transfer the cooked pasta back to the pot it was boiled in, and stir in half of the **Cauliflower Alfredo Sauce**. Add more sauce as desired and heat until warm, about 5 minutes.

4. To serve, transfer the pasta to plates and top it with the roasted vegetables.

CHICKPEA CRUST
rainbow alfredo PIZZA

⊕ **TOTAL TIME:** 40 MINUTES   **ACTIVE TIME:** 20 MINUTES   **MAKES:** 4 SERVINGS

What's more fun than pizza? A rainbow pizza on easy-to-make gluten-free crust! The crust is a variation on socca, an Italian chickpea-based flatbread. It's different than typical pizza crust, but it's equally delicious in its own way (thank you, Italian cuisine, for always hitting the high notes of deliciousness), especially when topped with a rainbow of veggies.

CHICKPEA CRUST
2 cups chickpea flour
1 cup water
1 tablespoon olive oil
Dash of salt

TOPPINGS
½ batch Cauliflower Alfredo
   Sauce (see page 239)
1 batch Rainbow Roasted
   Vegetables (see page 165)

1. To prepare the chickpea crust, preheat the oven to 375°F. Line a baking sheet with parchment paper.

2. In a medium bowl, whisk all the crust ingredients together until smooth. Use a spatula or spoon to spread the batter out on the baking sheet in a circular shape until it's about ¼ inch thick.

3. Bake for 15–20 minutes, until the edges are crisp. Remove from the oven, and gently flip the parchment paper and crust upside down on the baking sheet. Peel off the parchment paper.

4. Spread all but 2 tablespoons of the **Cauliflower Alfredo Sauce** over the crust. To make the presentation especially showstopping, arrange the rainbow roasted vegetables in rainbow order with the cherry tomatoes, carrots, yellow bell pepper, and broccoli followed by the red onion and purple cabbage. Drizzle the remaining 2 tablespoons of sauce on top.

5. Return to the oven and bake for about 10 minutes, until everything is warm. Slice and serve.

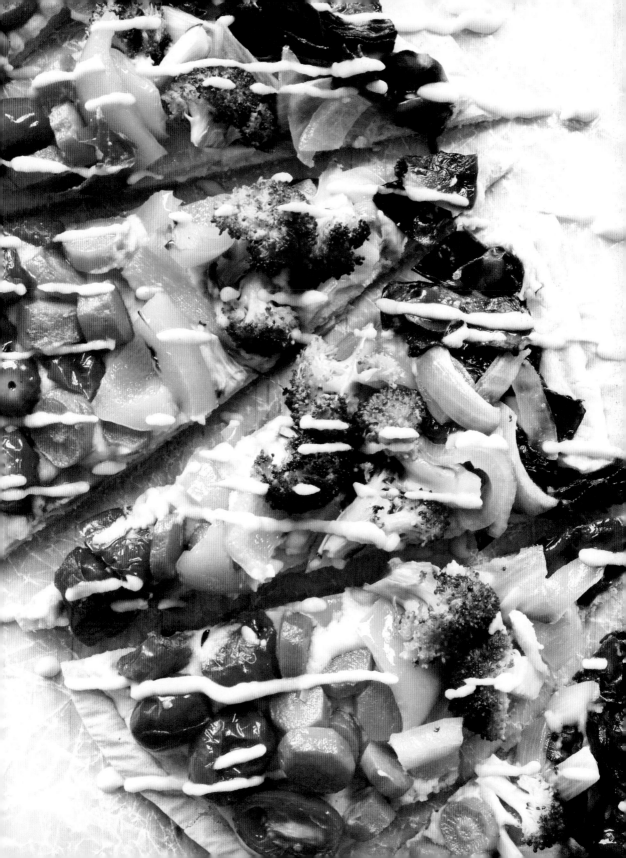

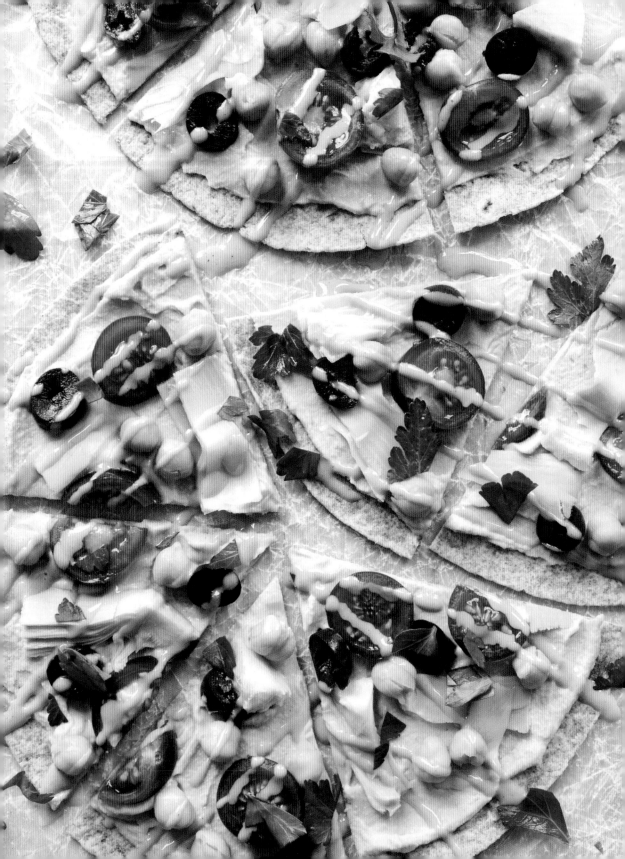

EASY HUMMUS & *artichoke* TORTILLA PIZZA

⊕ **TOTAL TIME:** 10 MINUTES **MAKES:** 4 SERVINGS

For nights when you really don't feel like cooking dinner, this simple pizza has your back.

---

4 large tortillas*

1 cup hummus, store-bought or homemade (see pages 122–124)

1½ cups cooked chickpeas (or one 15-ounce can, rinsed and drained)

1½ cups chopped artichoke hearts (or one 15-ounce can, drained and chopped)

1 cup cherry tomatoes, sliced in half

¼ cup sliced black olives

¼ cup tahini

2 tablespoons chopped fresh parsley

Salt and black pepper, to taste

1. Preheat the oven to 400°F.*

2. Place the tortillas on a baking sheet. Spread the hummus over the tortillas. Top with the chickpeas, artichoke hearts, cherry tomatoes, and olives.

3. Bake the tortillas until warm, 7–10 minutes.

4. Drizzle the tahini over the tortillas, and sprinkle with the parsley, salt, and pepper. Slice and enjoy right away.

NOTE: *I love the texture of brown rice tortillas, plus they're gluten-free.*

NOTE: *If you're feeling especially lazy, go ahead and serve this pizza cold. It's still great.*

BBQ RANCH
cauliflower PIZZA

⊕ **TOTAL TIME:** 20 MINUTES **ACTIVE TIME:** 10 MINUTES **MAKES:** 4 SERVINGS

Sports are just an excuse for snacks, right? My husband might disagree with me about that, but he definitely does agree that this fully loaded pizza is perfect for munching on while watching the big game.

1 prebaked pizza crust*
⅓ cup barbecue sauce
1 handful baby spinach
½ red onion, sliced
1 batch BBQ Cauliflower
   Poppers (see page 135)
½ cup shredded vegan
   mozzarella cheese
½ batch Green Cashew Ranch
   Dressing (see page 234)
2 tablespoons chopped
   fresh parsley

1. Preheat the oven to 375°F.

2. Place the prebaked crust on a pizza stone or baking sheet. Spread the barbecue sauce evenly on top. Layer the spinach, onion, **BBQ Cauliflower Poppers**, and cheese on top.

3. Bake for about 10 minutes, until the cheese is melted.

4. Drizzle the **Green Cashew Ranch Dressing** on top, and sprinkle with the parsley.

NOTE: *Or use the chickpea crust on page 166.*

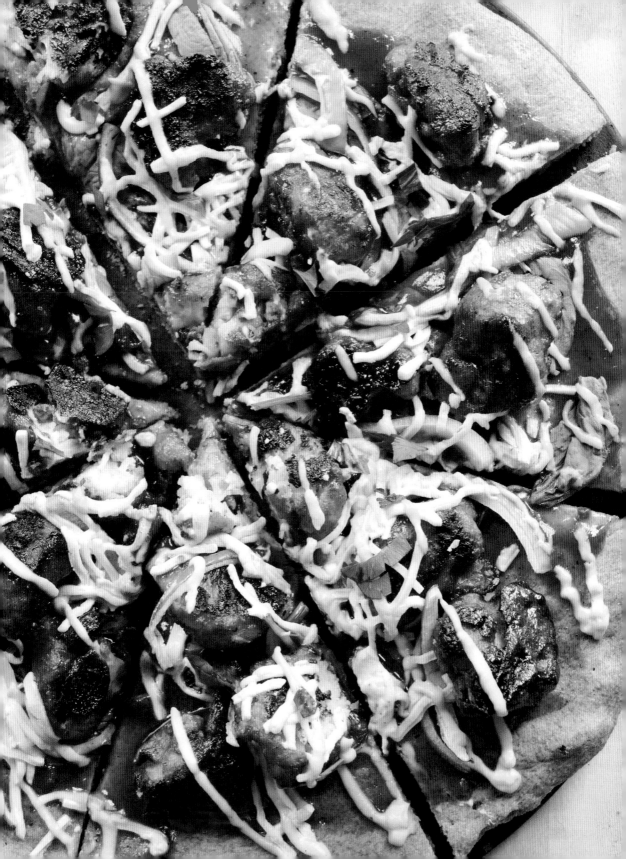

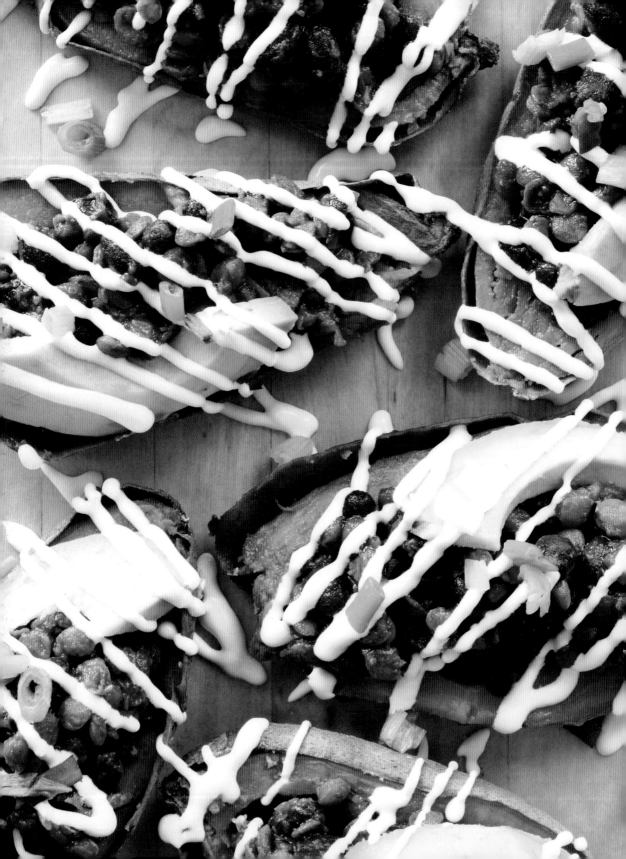

SWEET POTATO *skins*

⊕ **TOTAL TIME**: 1 HOUR 10 MINUTES **ACTIVE TIME**: 15 MINUTES **MAKES**: 4 SERVINGS

This is one of the very simple, staple recipes I keep in my "What's for dinner?" toolbox. Think of it as a blank canvas—you can easily jazz it up by adding just about any sauce from the Kitchen Staples & Sauces chapter (see page 221).

SWEET POTATO BASE
4 medium sweet potatoes
1 batch Lentils (see page 230)
1½ cups cooked black beans
   (or one 15-ounce can,
   rinsed and drained)
Salt and black pepper, to taste

TOPPINGS
1 avocado, sliced
Cashew Sour Cream (see
   page 226) or store-bought
   vegan sour cream
2 tablespoons chopped
   green onions
½ batch Green Tahini Sauce
   (see page 238), Miso-Ginger
   Sauce (see page 238), or
   whatever sauce you're in the
   mood for (optional)

1. To roast the sweet potatoes, preheat the oven to 400°F. Line a baking sheet with parchment paper. Use a knife to poke holes in the sweet potatoes, and place them on the baking sheet. Bake for 45–60 minutes, until tender. Remove the sweet potatoes from the oven, and let them sit until they are cool enough to handle.

2. While the sweet potatoes cool, combine the **Lentils** and black beans in a medium saucepan over medium-low heat. Heat them until warm, about 5 minutes. Season them with salt and pepper.

3. Slice the sweet potatoes in half lengthwise. Use a spoon to scoop out about half of the flesh from each. Reserve the scooped-out flesh for another use.* Spoon the lentil and black bean mixture into the sweet potatoes.

4. Top each sweet potato half with an avocado slice. Top with the **Cashew Sour Cream** and green onions. Add any sauce you like, if desired.

NOTE: *You can save the extra sweet potato flesh for **Savory Sweet Potato Toast** (see page 46).*

cheesy broccoli & BACON STUFFED POTATOES

⊕ **TOTAL TIME:** 1 HOUR 5 MINUTES **ACTIVE TIME:** 20 MINUTES **MAKES:** 4 SERVINGS

My best friend, Erica, and I used to have competitions for who could build the best potato at the make-your-own baked potato bar at our summer camp. We would pile our potatoes high, taste each other's to determine who dressed hers best, and then crown one of us the winner. Looking back, it was a rather strange way to spend our time at camp, but we considered it our favorite sport.

4 medium russet potatoes

1 broccoli crown, broken into florets (about 2 cups)

1 tablespoon olive oil

1 batch Cashew Cheese Sauce (see page 239)*

1 batch Tempeh Bacon (see page 231)

1 batch Cashew Sour Cream (see page 226) or store-bought vegan sour cream

2 tablespoons chopped green onions

Salt and black pepper, to taste

1. Preheat the oven to 400°F. Use a fork to poke holes in the potatoes. Place them on a baking sheet, and bake for about 1 hour, until the skin is crispy.

2. When the potatoes have about 15 minutes left to cook, toss the broccoli with the olive oil in a bowl. Spread out the broccoli on a second baking sheet. Bake the broccoli for about 15 minutes, flipping halfway through, until it's crispy.

3. Warm the **Cashew Cheese Sauce** in a small saucepan over low heat until the potatoes and broccoli are done baking.

4. Remove the potatoes and broccoli from the oven. Use a knife to slice the tops of the potatoes open. Stuff with the broccoli, **Tempeh Bacon**, and **Cashew Cheese Sauce**. Top everything with the warm **Cashew Sour Cream** and green onions, and sprinkle with salt and pepper.

NOTE: *For a little less prep work, you can skip the sauce and melt store-bought shredded vegan cheddar over everything.*

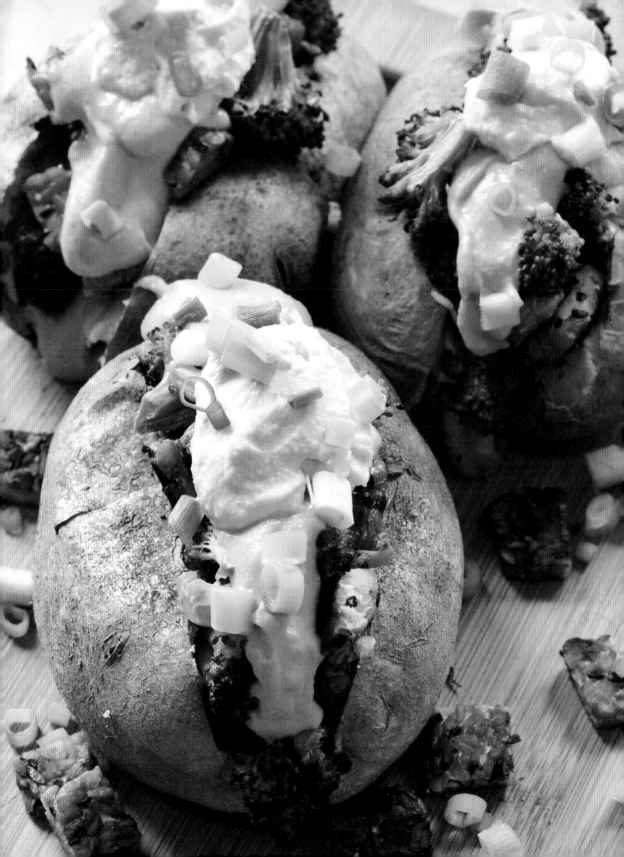

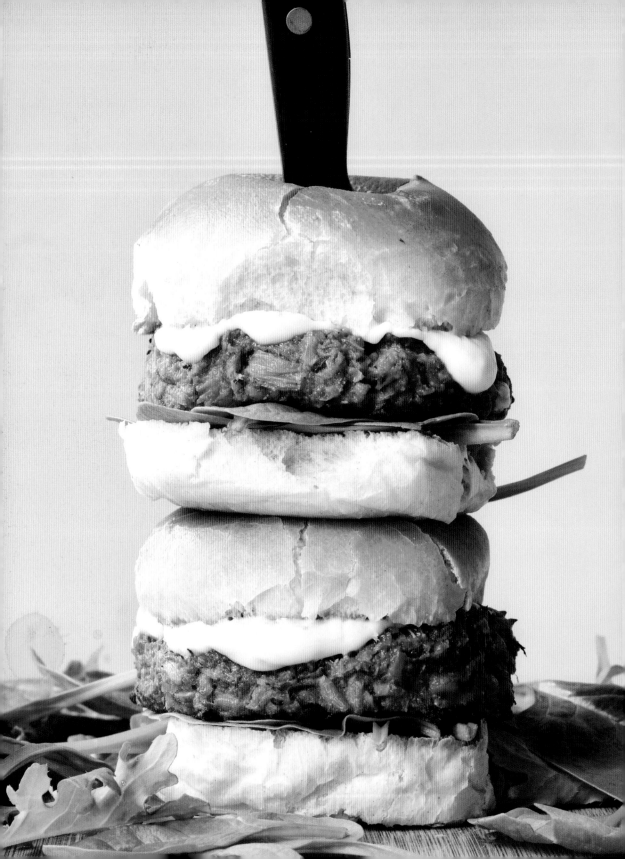

HARVEST BUTTERNUT SQUASH & APPLE *burger* WITH SAGE AIOLI

⊕ **TOTAL TIME:** 1 HOUR 20 MINUTES **ACTIVE TIME:** 30 MINUTES **MAKES:** 8–10 BURGERS

I've been known to go a little overboard on Thanksgiving recipes on my blog. From everything smothered in gravy to everything stuffed with pumpkin spice, I love the flavors of the fall season. These burgers offer a taste of my favorite holiday that you can enjoy all year long. They do take a bit of time to put together, so I like to make a double or triple batch and freeze these burgers for emergency T-Day cravings.

BURGERS
3 cups cubed butternut squash
2 tablespoons olive oil, divided
1 medium onion, diced
2 cloves garlic, minced
2 apples, peeled and diced
⅓ batch (about 1 cup) Brown Rice (see page 228)
1 tablespoon ground flaxseed
3 tablespoons warm water
1 tablespoon tamari
½ cup finely chopped walnuts
½ cup spelt flour
½ teaspoon dried rosemary
½ teaspoon dried thyme
½ teaspoon dried sage
Salt and black pepper, to taste

SAGE AIOLI
1 cup vegan mayo, store-bought or homemade (see page 224)
Juice of ½ lemon
4 cloves garlic, minced
2 tablespoons chopped fresh sage
Salt and black pepper, to taste

1. To prepare the burgers, preheat the oven to 400°F. Toss the squash cubes with 1 tablespoon of the olive oil, and spread them out on a baking sheet. Bake for 25 minutes, flipping halfway through.

2. While the squash cooks, heat the remaining 1 tablespoon olive oil in a medium pan over medium-high heat. Add the onion and garlic and sauté for 5 minutes. Turn the heat down to medium, add the apples and a splash of water, and cook until the apples are tender, about 10 minutes. Transfer the mixture to a large bowl.

3. When the squash is done roasting, remove it from the oven and turn the temperature down to 375°F. Transfer it to the bowl with the onion mixture and add the **Brown Rice**.

4. Prepare a flax "egg" by stirring the ground flaxseed and warm water together in a small bowl. Let the mixture sit for at least 10 minutes before using.

5. Use an immersion blender or a potato masher to blend all the ingredients in the large bowl together until a mushy texture is formed (some chunks are good). Stir in the flax "egg," tamari, walnuts, flour, rosemary, thyme, sage, salt, and pepper.

continued on next page...

ENTRÉES 177

6. Grease the baking sheet for the burgers. Wet your hands and form patties, using about ¾ cup of the mixture for each. There should be enough to make 8–10 burgers. Place them on the baking sheet. Bake for 20 minutes, then remove from the oven and flip the burgers. Return to the oven and bake for another 20 minutes, until the outsides are crispy.

7. While the burgers cook, prepare the sage aioli by whisking all the ingredients together. Store in the refrigerator until needed.

8. Serve the burgers warm on the buns, topped with the mixed greens and sage aioli.

BLACK BEAN BURGERS WITH *tahini-mustard* SLAW

⊕ **TOTAL TIME:** 1 HOUR 30 MINUTES **ACTIVE TIME:** 30 MINUTES **MAKES:** 8 BURGERS

I haven't always been a burger gal. It wasn't until I met my husband, who is very much a burger guy, that I began to appreciate the magic of a good burger. Watching him swoon over veggie ones at restaurants inspired me to come up with this recipe, which became an instant classic in our house. He describes this recipe as a "real meal"—so bring your appetite. This recipe is quite time-consuming, so always double or triple the batch and freeze some burgers for later on.

BURGERS
1 medium sweet potato*
1 tablespoon olive oil
1 small yellow onion, diced
2 cloves garlic, minced
1 tablespoon ground flaxseed
3 tablespoons warm water
⅓ batch (about 1 cup) Brown Rice (see page 228)
1½ cups black beans (or one 15-ounce can, rinsed and drained)
½ cup flour of your choice
1 tablespoon liquid smoke
1 tablespoon tamari
2 teaspoon vegan Worcestershire sauce
½ teaspoon smoked paprika
⅛ teaspoon salt
Dash of black pepper

TAHINI-MUSTARD SLAW
1 cup thinly sliced cabbage
1 tablespoon tahini
1 tablespoon Dijon mustard
2 teaspoons olive oil
2 teaspoons maple syrup
2 teaspoons tamari
Salt and black pepper, to taste

1. To prepare the burgers, preheat the oven to 400°F.

2. Use a knife to poke holes in the sweet potato, and place it on a baking sheet. Bake for 45–60 minutes, until tender. Remove the sweet potato from the oven, and let it sit until it is cool enough to handle. When it's cool, peel off the skin, scoop the flesh into a large bowl, and mash it with a fork.

3. Turn the oven down to 375°F.

4. In a small pan, heat the olive oil over medium-high heat. Add the yellow onion and garlic and sauté until browned, 7–10 minutes. Transfer to the bowl with the sweet potato.

5. Prepare a flax "egg" by stirring the ground flaxseed and warm water together in a small bowl. Let the mixture sit for at least 10 minutes before using.

6. Add the **Brown Rice** and black beans to the bowl with the sweet potato. Use an immersion blender or potato masher to mash together the mixture until it has a partially smooth texture.

7. Add the flour, liquid smoke, tamari, Worcestershire sauce, paprika, salt, pepper, and flax "egg" to the sweet potato mixture, and stir until thoroughly mixed.

continued on next page...

SERVE WITH
Burger buns
Tomato slices
Red onion slices
Your choice of condiments
   (ketchup, mustard, vegan
   mayo, etc.)

8. Grease a baking sheet. Wet your hands and form patties, using about ¾ cup of the mixture for each. There should be enough to make 8 burgers. Place them on the baking sheet.

9. Bake for 25 minutes, then remove from the oven and flip the burgers. Return to the oven and bake for another 15 minutes, until the outsides are crispy.

10. While the burgers bake, prepare the tahini-mustard slaw. Combine all the ingredients in a large bowl and stir together until the cabbage is thoroughly coated. Store in the refrigerator until ready to use.

11. Serve the burgers warm on the buns, topped with the slaw, tomato slices, red onion slices, and your favorite condiments. Refrigerate the burgers if you aren't eating them right away, or freeze them for up to 3 months.

NOTE: *As an alternative, you can use ¾ cup of sweet potato puree and skip steps 1 and 2.*

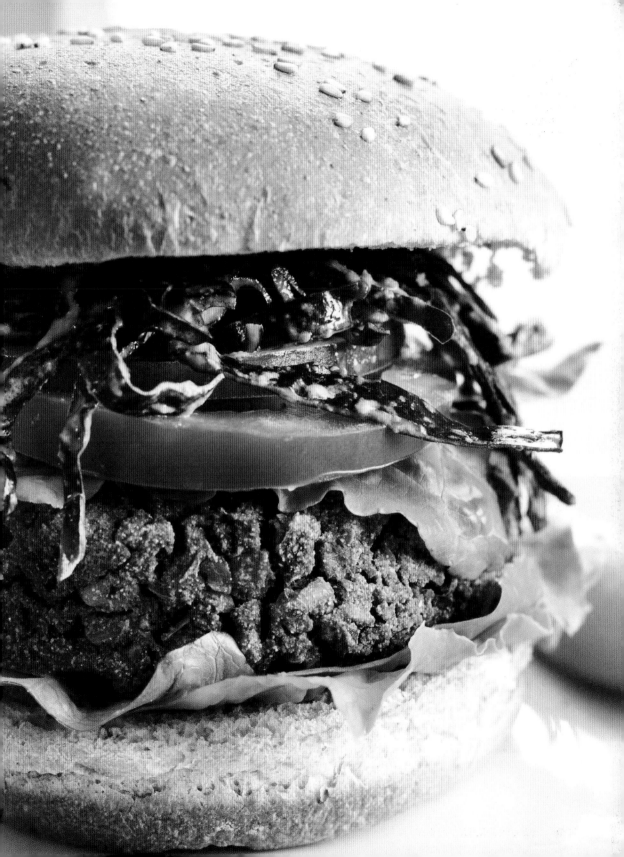

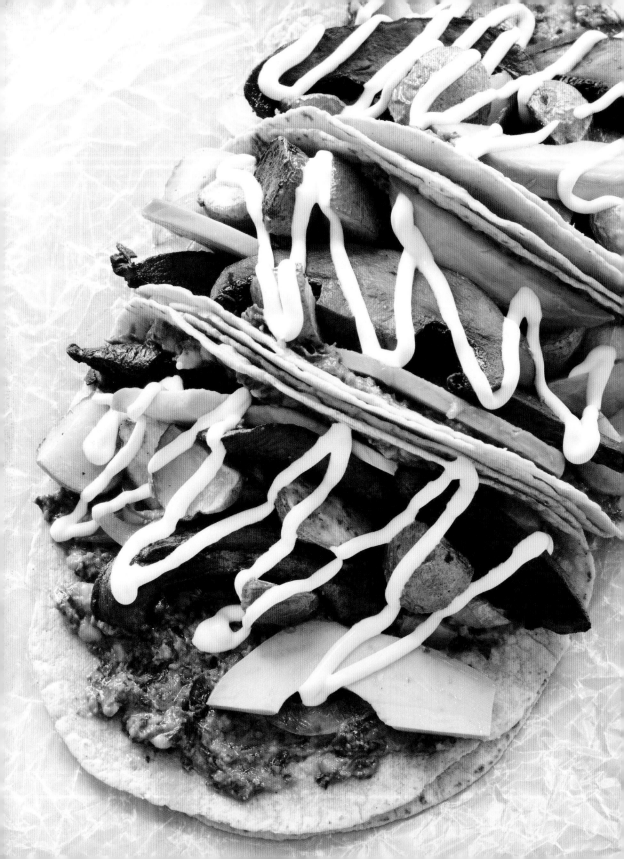

PORTOBELLO & POTATO *pesto* TACOS

TOTAL TIME: 35 MINUTES **ACTIVE TIME:** 10 MINUTES **MAKES:** 4 SERVINGS

Take Taco Tuesday to the next level with this recipe that's far from standard. These tacos start with a hearty base of roasted mushrooms and potatoes, and are perfectly balanced with light and fresh pesto, avocado slices, and Cashew Sour Cream. For extra protein, Baked Tofu (see page 233) or Tempeh Bacon (see page 231) are great additions.

4 portobello mushrooms, cut into ½-inch-thick slices
3 cups cubed red potatoes
1 medium onion, sliced
2 tablespoons olive oil
Salt and black pepper, to taste
8 small tortillas
1 batch Kale & Avocado Pesto (see page 236)
1 avocado, sliced
1 batch Cashew Sour Cream (see page 226) or store-bought vegan sour cream

1. Preheat the oven to 400°F.

2. In a large bowl, toss the mushrooms, potatoes, and onion with the olive oil. Spread the vegetables out on a baking sheet. Sprinkle with salt and pepper.

3. Bake for 15 minutes, flip the vegetables, then bake for 10 more minutes.

4. To assemble the tacos, spread the tortillas with the **Kale & Avocado Pesto**, and top with the baked vegetables, avocado, and **Cashew Sour Cream**. Serve immediately.

REUBEN-ISH *bowl*

⊕ **TOTAL TIME:** 10 MINUTES **MAKES:** 4 SERVINGS

A much healthier twist on the classic NYC deli sandwich, this recipe is a flavor party in a bowl. Double your ingredient prep and pack a Reuben-ish sandwich for lunch the next day. (Just prepare the Grilled Reuben-ish on page 106, but skip the grilling.)

1 batch cooked Brown Rice (see page 228)
6 cups packed baby spinach
1 batch Baked Tofu (see page 233), sliced
½ cup sauerkraut
½ cup sliced pickles
1 batch Thousand Island Dressing (see page 235)
Salt and black pepper, to taste

1. Divide the **Brown Rice** into 4 bowls.

2. To wilt the spinach, put it in a pan with a splash of water and cook it over medium heat. Stir for about 2 minutes, until the spinach wilts. Spoon the spinach over the rice in the bowls.

3. Layer the **Baked Tofu**, sauerkraut, and pickles over the spinach. Drizzle the **Thousand Island Dressing** on top, and sprinkle with salt and pepper.

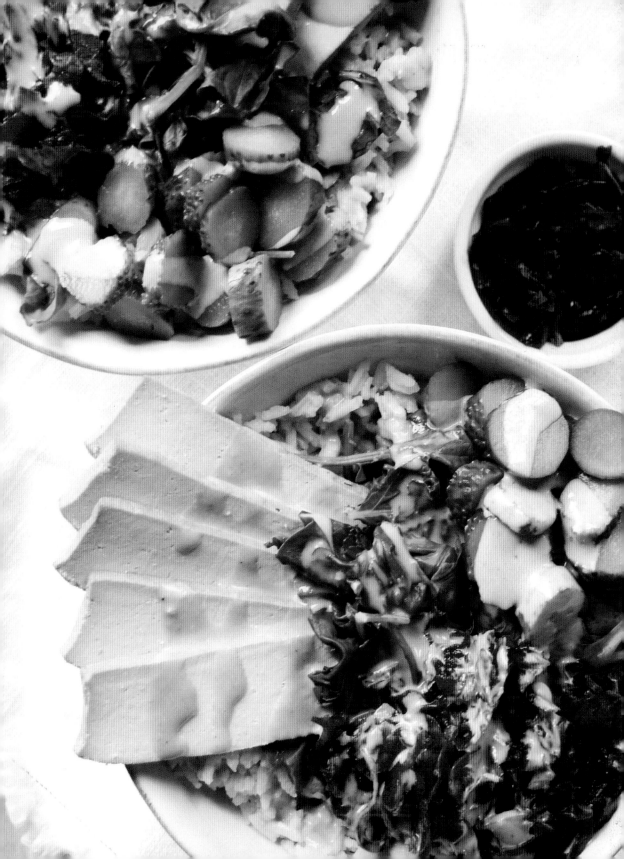

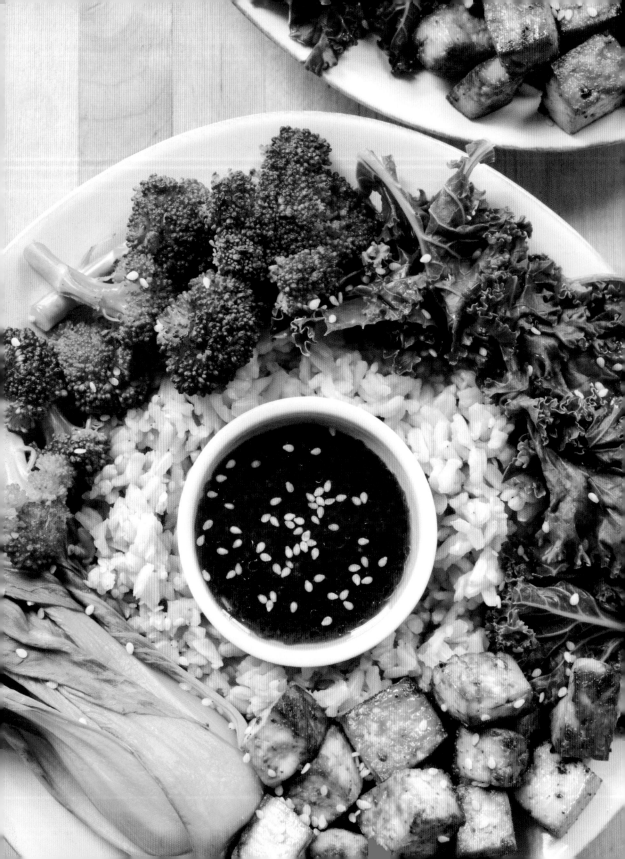

STEEMED GREENS & *tofu bowl* WITH MISO-GINGER SAUCE

⊕ **TOTAL TIME:** 10 MINUTES **MAKES:** 4 SERVINGS

Since my first foray into wholesome eating was through the macrobiotic diet (see page 11), macro bowls always help me reset back to my healthy place. This is one of my favorite versions to make for rainy-day lunches or dinner at the end of an exhausting day, when I need something extra nourishing to boost me back up.

1 broccoli crown, broken into
   florets (about 2 cups)
4 heads baby bok choy, ends
   cut off
1 bunch kale, chopped
1 batch Brown Rice (see
   page 228)
1 batch Baked Tofu (see
   page 233), cut into cubes
1 batch Miso-Ginger Sauce
   (see page 238)
1 tablespoon sesame seeds

1. Bring a pot of water to a boil over high heat. Put the broccoli in a steamer basket on top of the pot, cover, and steam for 5 minutes, until it turns bright green.

2. Add the bok choy and steam for another 2 minutes. Add the kale and steam for another 3 minutes.

3. Divide the **Brown Rice** into 4 bowls and layer the steamed vegetables on top. Add the **Baked Tofu** and **Miso-Ginger Sauce**. Top with the sesame seeds and serve immediately.

MAPLE-MUSTARD SQUASH & *lentil* BOWL

⊕ **TOTAL TIME:** 1 HOUR **ACTIVE TIME:** 20 MINUTES **MAKES:** 4 SERVINGS

A slightly jazzed-up take on the traditional macro bowl, this hearty and filling recipe features kabocha squash, which is one of the most naturally sweet varieties of squash. When roasted, it becomes extra tender and simply melts in your mouth. I could go on about this squash all day, but if you can't find it at your local grocery store or farmer's market, any variety of squash (butternut, acorn, and so on) will still be delicious. Consider doubling up on the roasted squash to whip up Maple-Mustard Squash Grilled Cheese (see page 113) the next day.

1 medium kabocha squash, peeled if desired
1 batch Maple-Mustard Sauce (see page 237)
1 broccoli crown, broken into florets (about 2 cups)
1 pound baby spinach
1 batch Lentils (see page 230)
1½ cups cooked black beans (or one 15-ounce can, rinsed and drained)
¼ cup sauerkraut
1 avocado, sliced

1. To prepare the roasted squash, preheat the oven to 400°F. Slice the squash in half, scoop out the seeds, and cut it into slices ½ to ¾ inch thick. Place the slices in a large bowl.

2. Toss the squash with half of the **Maple-Mustard Sauce.** Spread the squash out on a baking sheet. Bake for 45 minutes, flipping halfway through.

3. For the steamed vegetables, bring a pot of water to a boil over high heat. Put the broccoli in a steamer basket on top of the pot, cover, and steam for 5 minutes, until it turns bright green.

4. Add the spinach and steam for another 1–2 minutes, until it wilts.

5. Divide the **Lentils** into 4 bowls and layer the roasted squash, black beans, sauerkraut, avocado, and steamed broccoli and spinach on top. Drizzle the rest of the **Maple-Mustard Sauce** on top.

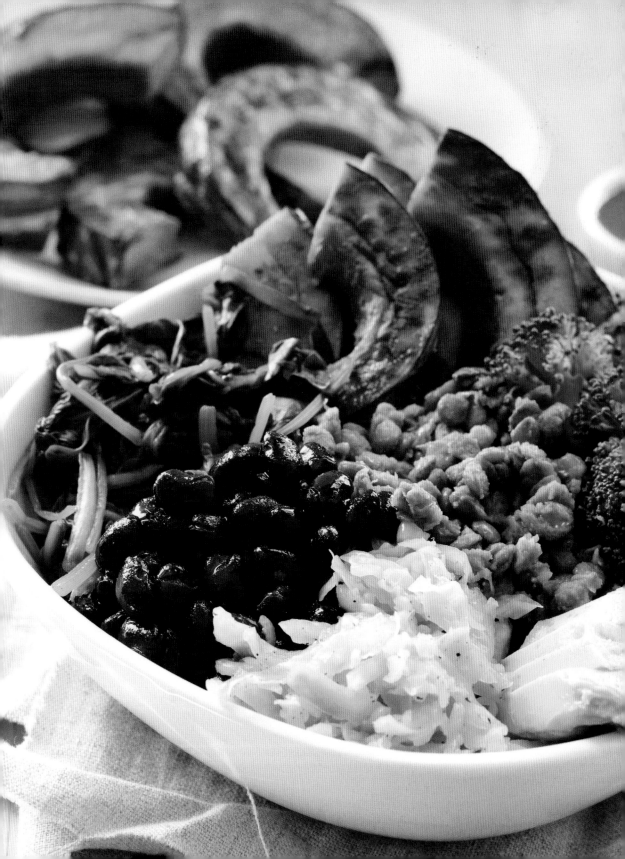

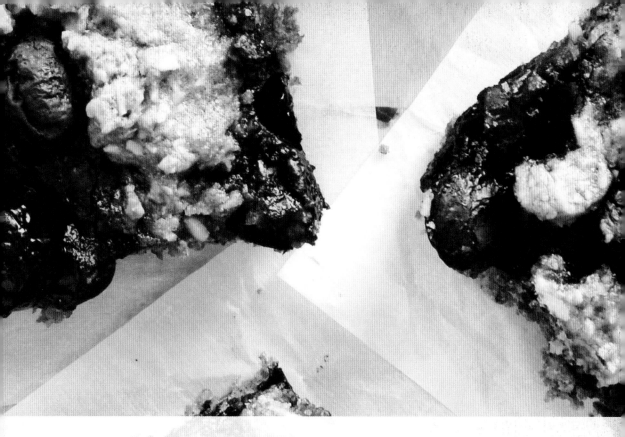

dessert

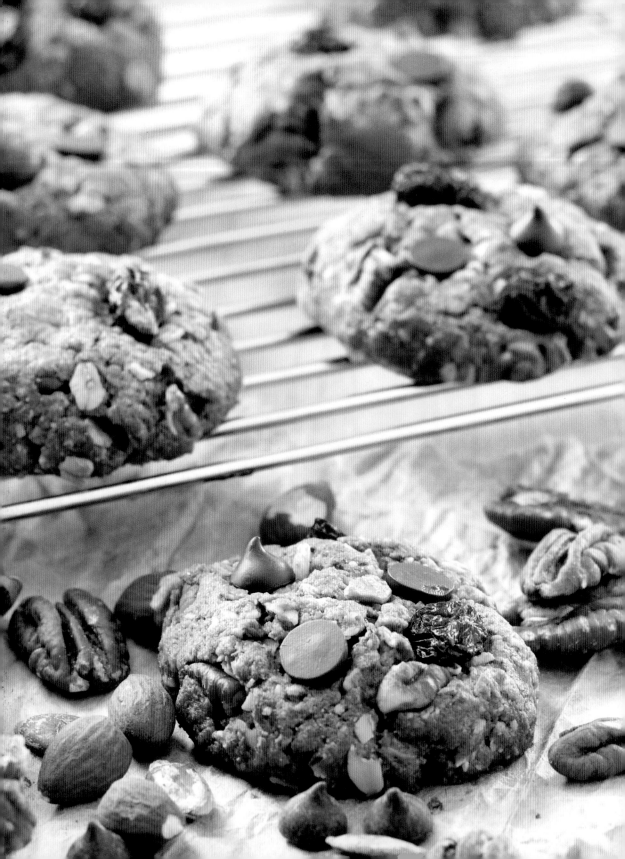

trail mix OATMEAL COOKIES

TOTAL TIME: 25 MINUTES   **ACTIVE TIME:** 15 MINUTES   **MAKES:** ABOUT 20 COOKIES

You know when it's 3 PM, you're starting to feel sluggish, and you kind of want to face-plant into a bathtub of coffee? Try these protein-and-fiber-filled cookies to perk you up instead.

FLAX "EGG"
1 tablespoon ground flaxseed
3 tablespoons warm water

DRY
1 cup spelt flour
1 cup rolled oats
⅔ cup coconut sugar
½ cup chopped walnuts, almonds, pumpkin seeds, and sunflower seeds*
½ teaspoon baking soda
¼ teaspoon salt

WET
⅓ cup coconut oil, melted
⅓ cup peanut butter
¼ cup nondairy milk
2 teaspoons vanilla extract

FOLD-INS
⅓ cup raisins
⅓ cup chocolate chips

1. Preheat the oven to 350°F. Grease a baking sheet or line it with parchment paper.

2. Prepare the flax "egg" by stirring the ground flaxseed and warm water together in a small bowl. Let the mixture sit for at least 10 minutes before using.

3. In a large bowl, whisk the dry ingredients together.

4. In a small bowl, stir the wet ingredients together until smooth. Add the flax "egg" and stir again. Transfer the contents of the small bowl to the large bowl, and mix until the wet and dry ingredients are thoroughly combined. Fold in the raisins and chocolate chips.

5. Spoon out balls of dough, a little more than 1 tablespoon each, and place them on the baking sheet. Use your hand or the back of a spoon to slightly flatten each ball.

6. Bake for 11–13 minutes, until the edges are slightly golden. Remove from the oven and transfer the cookies to a cooling rack. Let them cool completely, then enjoy right away or store in an airtight container.

NOTE: *This is my favorite mix of nuts and seeds, but go crazy with your favorite combination.*

PB&J *thumbprint* COOKIES

TOTAL TIME: 30 MINUTES **ACTIVE TIME:** 15 MINUTES **MAKES:** ABOUT 14 COOKIES

This no-fuss recipe is one of my favorites for weeknight baking. Keep it classic or get creative with different nut butters and fruit preserves—cashew butter and blueberry, almond butter and apricot—you can't go wrong.

DRY
1 cup rolled oats
¼ teaspoon baking soda
⅛ teaspoon salt

WET
½ cup creamy peanut butter
¼ cup maple syrup
2 tablespoons coconut oil, melted
1 teaspoon vanilla extract

TOPPINGS
½ cup jam or fruit preserves
2 tablespoons creamy peanut butter

1. Preheat the oven to 350°F. Grease a baking sheet or line it with parchment paper.

2. In a blender, pulse the oats until flour is formed, then transfer it to a large bowl. Whisk in the baking soda and salt.

3. In a small bowl, stir the wet ingredients together until smooth. Transfer the mixture to the large bowl, and stir until the wet and dry ingredients are thoroughly combined.

4. To form the cookies, use your hands to roll about 1 tablespoon of batter into a ball. Press it down on the baking sheet and use your thumb to create an indent in the center. Fill the center with the jam or preserves. Repeat until all the dough is used.

5. Bake for 12 minutes. Remove from the oven and transfer the cookies to a cooling rack. Let them cool completely, then drizzle with the peanut butter (you may want to use a pastry bag or a plastic baggie with a corner cut off for this). Enjoy right away or store in an airtight container.

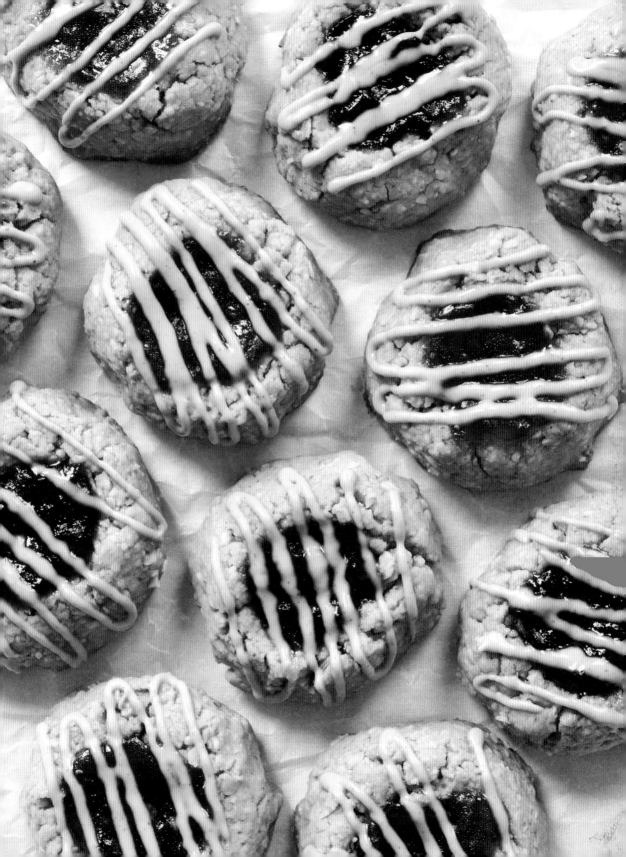

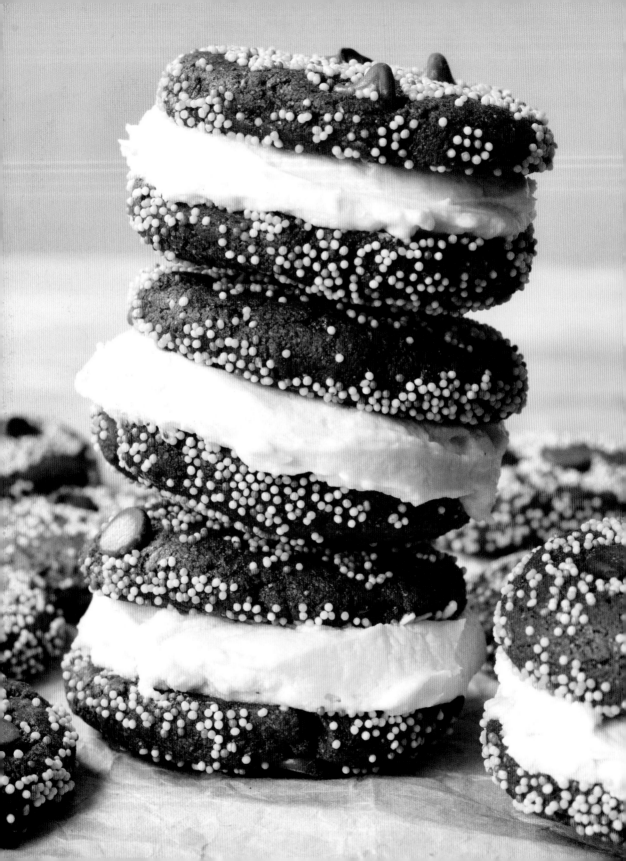

CHOCOLATE *cookie* SANDWICHES

⊕ **TOTAL TIME:** 35 MINUTES **ACTIVE TIME:** 20 MINUTES **MAKES:** 14 COOKIE SANDWICHES

These cookie sandwiches are totally decadent and made for frosting lovers. I couldn't decide if they taste better with vanilla or peanut butter frosting, so pick your favorite (or do half of each).

FLAX "EGG"
1 tablespoon ground flaxseed
3 tablespoons warm water

DRY
2 cups spelt flour
1 cup coconut sugar
½ cup cocoa powder
½ teaspoon baking soda
½ teaspoon baking powder
¼ teaspoon salt

WET
⅔ cup vegan butter or coconut oil, softened
½ cup nondairy milk
2 teaspoons vanilla extract

FOLD-INS
½ cup chocolate chips
Vegan sprinkles

FROSTING OPTIONS
1 batch Vanilla Frosting (see page 209)
1 batch Peanut Butter Frosting (see page 210)

1. Preheat the oven to 350°F. Grease a baking sheet or line it with parchment paper.

2. Prepare the flax "egg" by stirring together the ground flaxseed and warm water in a small bowl. Let the mixture sit for at least 10 minutes before using.

3. In a large bowl, whisk the dry ingredients together.

4. In a small bowl, stir the wet ingredients together until smooth. Add the flax "egg" and stir again. Transfer the contents of the small bowl to the large bowl, and mix until the wet and dry ingredients are thoroughly combined. Fold in the chocolate chips.

5. Wet your hands and roll a little more than 1 tablespoon of batter into a ball. Place it on the baking sheet and use your hand to slightly flatten it. Repeat until all the batter is used. Add the sprinkles on top.

6. Bake for 13 minutes. Remove from the oven and transfer the cookies to a cooling rack. Let them cool completely, then layer half of the cookies with the frosting of your choice, and top with the remaining cookies to make sandwiches. Enjoy right away or store in an airtight container in the refrigerator.

miso-tahini COOKIES

TOTAL TIME: 40 MINUTES **ACTIVE TIME:** 20 MINUTES **MAKES:** 20–24 COOKIES

These cookies are a favorite when I'm in the mood for something a bit savory and a bit sweet but not too sweet. When I was a pregnant lady, that mood escalated to a 24/7 craving, and I had to make these cookies every week.

FLAX "EGG"
1 tablespoon ground flaxseed
3 tablespoons warm water

DRY
1½ cups spelt flour
⅔ cup coconut sugar
½ teaspoon baking soda

WET
⅓ vegan butter or coconut oil, softened
⅓ cup tahini
3 tablespoons miso paste
6 tablespoons nondairy milk

COATING
½ cup chocolate chips
Sesame seeds

1. Preheat the oven to 350°F. Grease a baking sheet or line it with parchment paper.

2. Prepare the flax "egg" by stirring the ground flaxseed and warm water together in a small bowl. Let the mixture sit for at least 10 minutes before using.

3. In a large bowl, whisk the dry ingredients together.

4. In a small bowl, stir the wet ingredients together until smooth. Add the flax "egg" and stir again. Transfer the contents of the small bowl to the large bowl, and mix until the wet and dry ingredients are thoroughly combined.

5. Wet your hands and roll a little more than 1 tablespoon of batter into a ball. Place it on the baking sheet and use your hand to slightly flatten it. Repeat until all the batter is used.

6. Bake for 12 minutes. Remove from the oven and transfer the cookies to a cooling rack. Let them cool completely.

7. For the coating, line another baking sheet with wax paper. In a small saucepan, heat the chocolate chips over low heat and stir until melted, 3–4 minutes. Dip a cookie halfway into the chocolate. Place it on the baking sheet and sprinkle the chocolate coating with sesame seeds. Repeat with the rest of the cookies. Place the baking sheet in the refrigerator for 20–30 minutes to harden the chocolate before enjoying. Store the cookies in an airtight container.

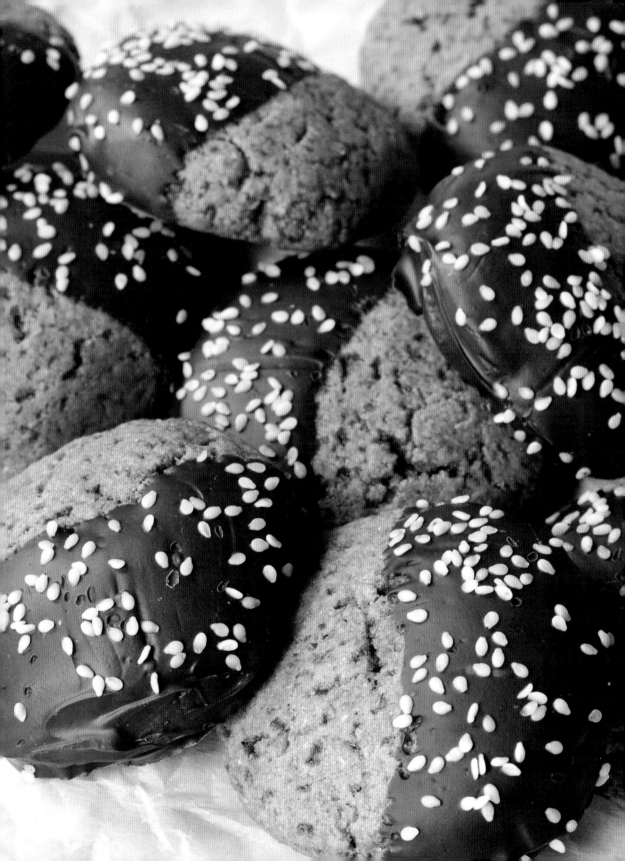

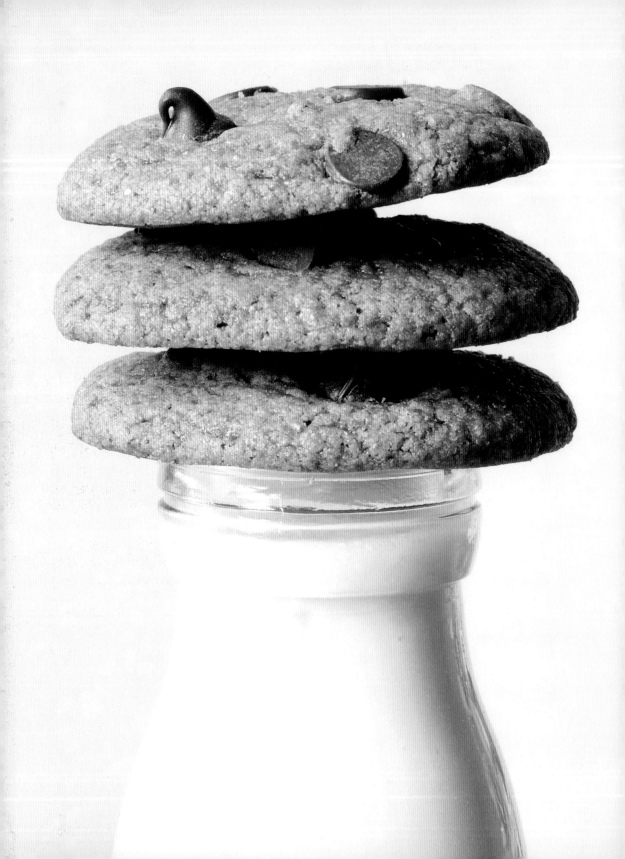

CLASSIC *chocolate chip* COOKIES

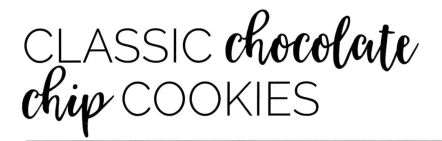

TOTAL TIME: 30 MINUTES **ACTIVE TIME:** 15 MINUTES **MAKES:** ABOUT 24 COOKIES

I came up with this recipe the week before my wedding, when life was super-chaotic and I was craving a simple, homey flavor from my childhood. These cookies taste like the ones we used to make that come out of a tube, but with a major ingredient upgrade.

FLAX "EGG"
1 tablespoon ground flaxseed
3 tablespoons warm water

DRY
2 cups spelt flour
⅔ cup coconut sugar
½ teaspoon baking soda
⅛ teaspoon salt

WET
⅔ cup vegan butter or
   coconut oil, softened
¼ cup nondairy milk
2 teaspoons vanilla extract

FOLD-IN
½ cup chocolate chips

1. Preheat the oven to 350°F. Grease a baking sheet or line it with parchment paper.

2. Prepare the flax "egg" by stirring the ground flaxseed and warm water together in a small bowl. Let the mixture sit for at least 10 minutes before using.

3. In a large bowl, whisk the dry ingredients together.

4. In a small bowl, stir the wet ingredients together until smooth. Add the flax "egg" and stir again. Transfer the contents of the small bowl to the large bowl, and mix until the wet and dry ingredients are thoroughly combined. Fold in the chocolate chips.

5. Spoon out balls of dough, a little more than 1 tablespoon each, and place them on the baking sheet. Use your hand to slightly flatten each scoop.

6. Bake for 11–13 minutes, until the edges are lightly golden. Remove from the oven and transfer the cookies to a cooling rack. Let them cool or dig in while warm. Store in an airtight container.

CHOCOLATE MOUSSE
cookie crumble PARFAIT

⊕ **TOTAL TIME:** 15 MINUTES (PLUS TIME FOR CHILLING COCONUT MILK) **MAKES:** 8 PARFAITS

Can we take a moment to appreciate the magic of coconut cream? It's the secret ingredient in this light and fluffy chocolate mousse, which couldn't be easier to make. I can eat spoonfuls of the mousse on its own, but it's even more perfect when paired with cookie crumbles in this parfait.

2 (13½-ounce) cans full-fat coconut milk, chilled in refrigerator at least 8 hours

¼ cup cocoa powder

¼ cup maple syrup

Dash of salt

½ batch Classic Chocolate Chip Cookies (see page 201), crumbled

1. To prepare the chocolate mousse, open the cans of coconut milk, drain the liquid on top (or save it for a smoothie), and scoop out the cream. Put the cream in a blender or a bowl with an electric mixer, and add the cocoa powder, maple syrup, and salt. Blend until smooth. Store in the refrigerator if not using right away.

2. Divide half of the crumbled **Classic Chocolate Chip Cookies** into 8 parfait glasses. Top each with 2–3 tablespoons of the chocolate mousse, and then add another layer of cookie crumbles on top. Serve immediately.

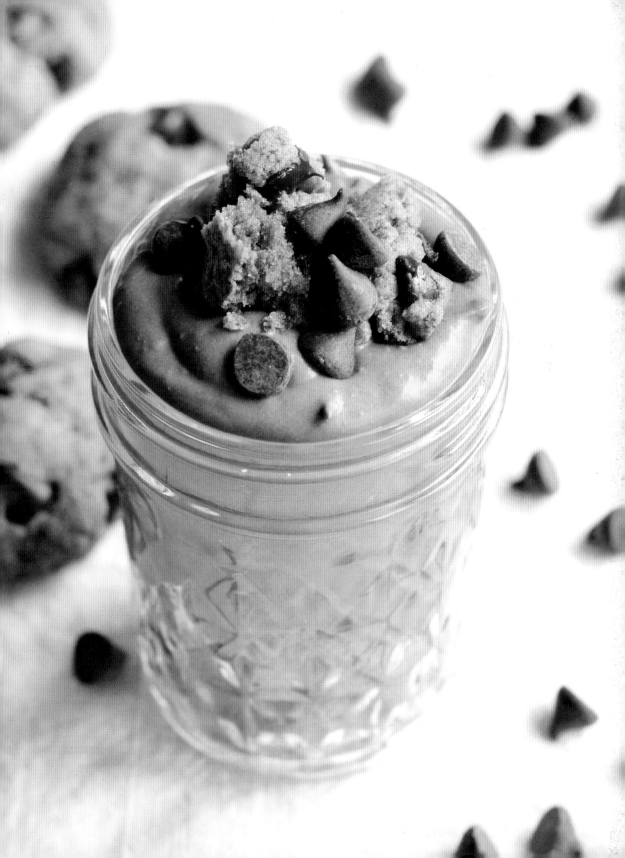

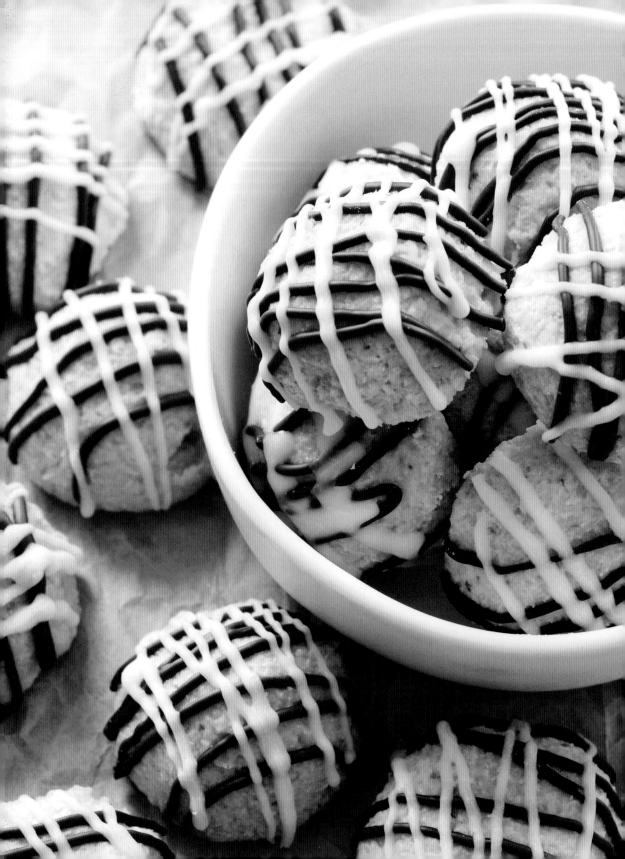

NO-BAKE *strawberry* MACAROONS

TOTAL TIME: 30 MINUTES   **ACTIVE TIME:** 20 MINUTES   **MAKES:** ABOUT 16 MACAROONS

This is a fun recipe because friends who try it can never believe how short the ingredient list is! I love to make these macaroons during the summer when strawberries are in season and I'm craving a light and fresh dessert.

MACAROONS
1½ cups shredded coconut
⅓ cup coconut butter, softened
½ cup chopped strawberries
¼ cup maple syrup
½ teaspoon vanilla extract
Dash of salt

DRIZZLE
¼ cup chocolate chips
¼ cup coconut butter, softened*

1. Line a baking sheet with parchment paper.

2. To prepare the macaroons, combine all the macaroon ingredients in a blender or food processor. Blend until mostly smooth, leaving a slightly grainy texture.

3. Wet your hands and roll a little more than 1 tablespoon of batter into a ball. Place it on the baking sheet and use your hand to slightly flatten it. Repeat until all the batter is used. Place the baking sheet in the freezer for 15 minutes to set.

4. For the chocolate drizzle, melt the chocolate chips in a small saucepan over low heat, stirring occasionally for 3–4 minutes, until melted. Use a spoon to drizzle the melted chocolate over the macaroons or use a pastry bag (or a plastic baggie with a corner cut off).

5. For the coconut butter drizzle, use a spoon or pastry bag to drizzle it over the macaroons.

6. Return the macaroons to the freezer for 5 minutes to set. Enjoy right away or store in an airtight container in the refrigerator.

NOTE: *To soften the coconut butter, place the jar in a bowl of hot water for 5 minutes before measuring it out.*

NO-BAKE STRAWBERRY
cheesecake

⊕ **TOTAL TIME:** 20 MINUTES (PLUS TIME FOR SOAKING CASHEWS AND CHILLING)
MAKES: 1 CHEESECAKE (8–10 SERVINGS)

This is one of my favorite desserts to make for birthdays or summer parties. Even though it requires a bit of time and advance preparation, it's still quite easy to make—not to mention that it's totally delicious and wholesome.

CRUST
1 cup rolled oats
8–10 Medjool dates
    (depending on size), pitted*
½ cup chopped walnuts
3 tablespoons coconut oil,
    softened
Dash of salt

FILLING
3 cups raw cashews, soaked
    in water at least 4 hours
2 cups chopped strawberries
½ cup maple syrup
⅓ cup coconut oil, softened
Juice of 3 lemons
1 tablespoon vanilla extract
Dash of salt

TOPPINGS
1 batch Coconut Whipped
    Cream (see page 227)
Whole or sliced strawberries

1. To prepare the crust, pulse the oats in a blender or food processor until a flour is formed. Add the dates, walnuts, coconut oil, and salt, and blend until a mostly smooth texture is formed.

2. Roll the mixture into a ball and use your hands to press it firmly down in the bottom of a 9-inch springform pan. Place the pan in the refrigerator to set while you prepare the filling.

3. To prepare the filling, drain the cashews and transfer them to a blender or food processor. Add the strawberries, maple syrup, coconut oil, lemon juice, vanilla extract, and salt, and blend until completely smooth (you'll need to scrape the sides down a few times).

4. Remove the springform pan from the refrigerator. Pour the filling into the pan, using a spatula to spread it out evenly. Place the cheesecake in the refrigerator to set for at least 4 hours (overnight is great) or in the freezer for 2 hours. When the cheesecake is firm, remove it from the springform pan and top it with the **Coconut Whipped Cream** and strawberries. Store it in the refrigerator until you're ready to enjoy it.

NOTE: *If you aren't using a high-speed blender, you may want to soften the dates by soaking them in hot water for 5 minutes so they blend smoothly.*

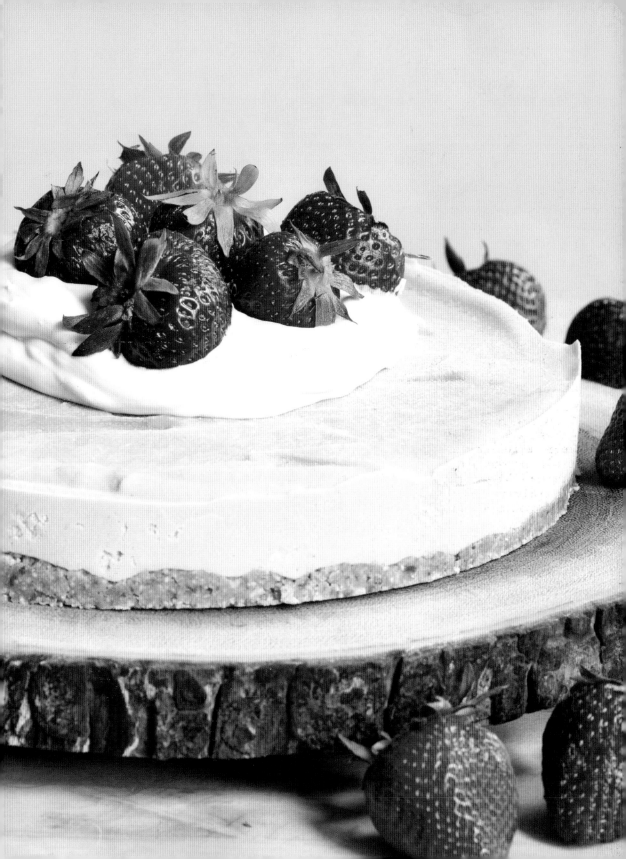

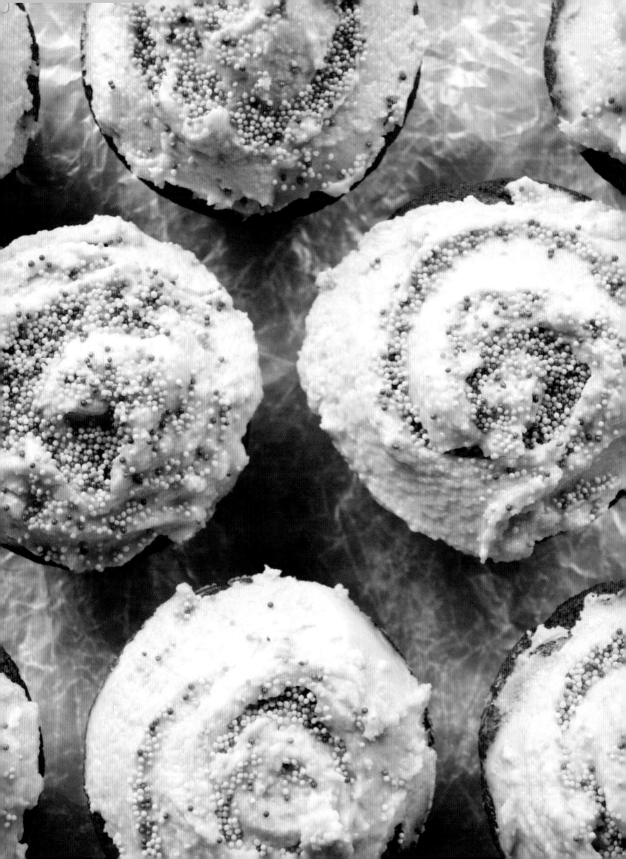

VERY *vanilla* CUPCAKES

TOTAL TIME: 55 MINUTES **ACTIVE TIME:** 15 MINUTES **MAKES:** 12 CUPCAKES

Wasn't it just the most exciting thing ever when someone would bring cupcakes to school on their birthday? This recipe is a throwback to the vanilla-on-vanilla childhood birthday fun.

VEGAN "BUTTERMILK"
1 cup nondairy milk
1 teaspoon apple cider vinegar

DRY
2 cups spelt flour
1 cup coconut sugar
1½ teaspoons baking powder
½ teaspoon baking soda
¼ teaspoon salt

WET
½ cup vegan butter or coconut oil, melted
1 tablespoon vanilla extract

VANILLA FROSTING
3 cups powdered sugar
1 cup vegan butter
1 teaspoon vanilla extract
Splash of nondairy milk, as needed to blend

TOPPING
Vegan sprinkles

1. Preheat the oven to 350°F. Grease a muffin tin or line it with baking cups.

2. In a small bowl, stir the nondairy milk and apple cider vinegar together to create vegan "buttermilk." Let the mixture sit for at least 10 minutes.

3. In a large bowl, whisk the dry ingredients together.

4. Stir the wet ingredients into the small bowl with the "buttermilk" mixture. Transfer the contents of the small bowl to the large bowl, and mix until the wet and dry ingredients are smooth.

5. Spoon the batter into the muffin wells, until each is about three-quarters full. Bake for 25 minutes, until lightly golden.

6. While the cupcakes bake, prepare the vanilla frosting by combining all the frosting ingredients together in a blender or in a bowl with an electric mixer.

7. Remove the cupcakes from the oven and transfer them to a cooling rack. Let them cool completely, then top them with the frosting and sprinkles and serve or store in an airtight container.

CHOCOLATE MINI CUPCAKES WITH *peanut butter* FROSTING

TOTAL TIME: 50 MINUTES   **ACTIVE TIME:** 15 MINUTES   **MAKES:** 40 MINI CUPCAKES

The only thing more fun than a cupcake is a mini cupcake. Each one of these little guys is like a bite-size party. If you love peanut butter, you'll go nuts for this extra-indulgent peanut butter frosting.

VEGAN "BUTTERMILK"
1 cup nondairy milk
1 teaspoon apple cider vinegar

DRY
2 cups spelt flour
1 cup coconut sugar
¼ cup cocoa powder
1½ teaspoons baking powder
½ teaspoon baking soda
¼ teaspoon salt

WET
½ cup vegan butter or
  coconut oil, melted
1 tablespoon vanilla extract

FOLD-IN
½ cup chocolate chips

PEANUT BUTTER FROSTING
3 cups powdered sugar
½ cup vegan butter
½ cup peanut butter
1 teaspoon vanilla extract
Splash of nondairy milk, as
  needed to blend

1. Preheat the oven to 350°F. Grease two 24-cup mini muffin tins (40 muffin wells) or line them with baking cups.

2. In a small bowl, stir the nondairy milk and apple cider vinegar together to create vegan "buttermilk." Let the mixture sit for at least 10 minutes.

3. In a large bowl, whisk the dry ingredients together.

4. Stir the wet ingredients into the small bowl with the "buttermilk" mixture. Transfer the contents of the small bowl to the large bowl, and stir until the wet and dry ingredients are smooth. Fold in the chocolate chips.

5. Spoon the batter into the muffin wells, until each is about three-quarters full. Bake for 20 minutes.

6. While the cupcakes bake, prepare the peanut butter frosting by combining all the frosting ingredients together in a blender or in a bowl with an electric mixer.

7. Remove the cupcakes from the oven and transfer them to a cooling rack. Let them cool completely, then top them with the frosting and serve or store in an airtight container.

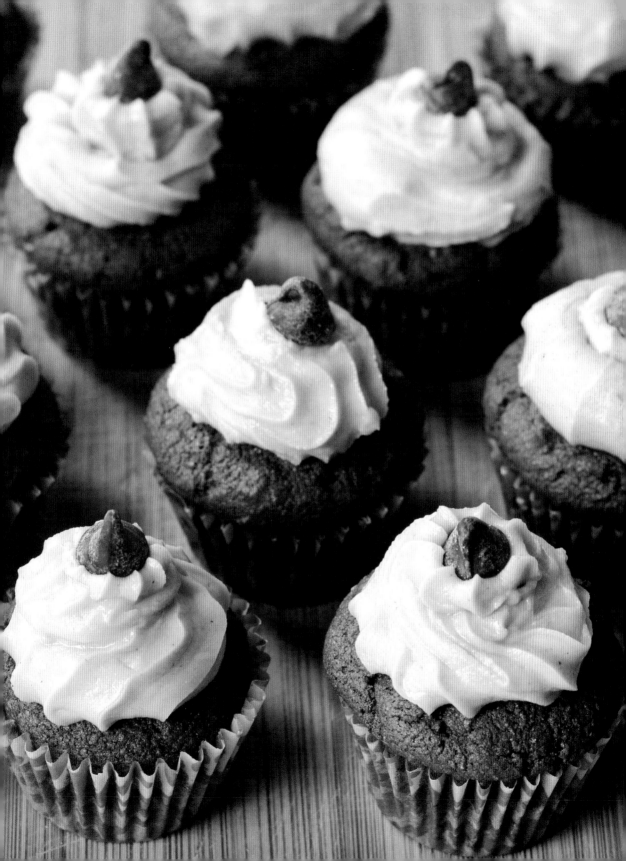

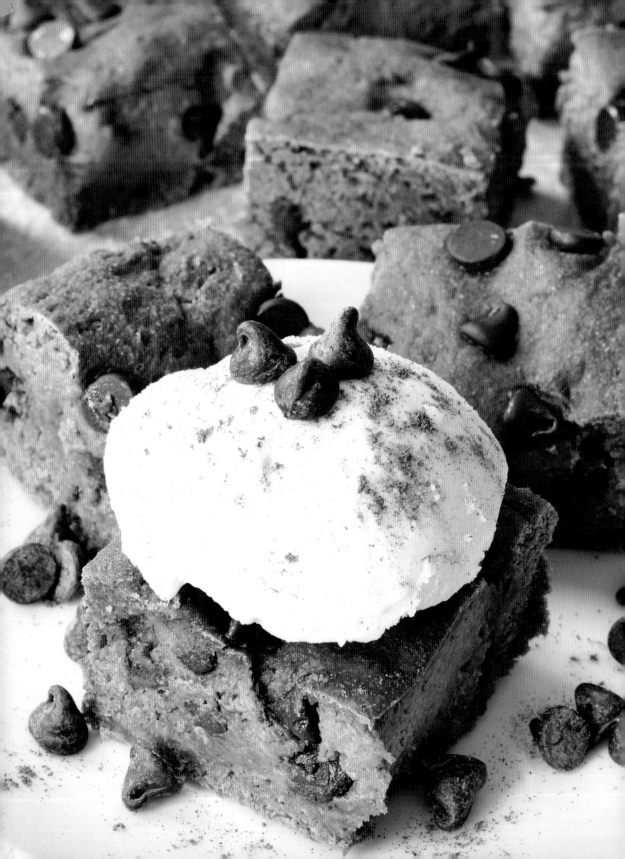

PUMPKIN SPICE
cake BARS

TOTAL TIME: 30 MINUTES   **ACTIVE TIME:** 10 MINUTES   **MAKES:** 12 BARS

I don't have a fireplace, but if I did I would enjoy this treat in front of a crackling fire, with my slippers on and mug of warm cider in one hand.

DRY
1½ cups spelt flour
½ cup coconut sugar
1 tablespoon pumpkin
  pie spice
½ teaspoon baking soda
¼ teaspoon salt

WET
1½ cups pumpkin puree
  (or one 15-ounce can)
¼ cup coconut oil, melted
¼ cup nondairy milk
1 tablespoon vanilla extract

FOLD-IN
½ cup chocolate chips

SERVE WITH
Store-bought vanilla nondairy
  ice cream

1. Preheat the oven to 375°F. Grease an 8-by-8-inch glass baking dish.

2. In a large bowl, whisk the dry ingredients together. In a small bowl, stir the wet ingredients together.

3. Stir the contents of the small bowl into the large bowl, and mix until the wet and dry ingredients are thoroughly combined. Fold in the chocolate chips. Transfer the batter to the baking dish and use a spatula to spread it out evenly.

4. Bake for 18 minutes, until golden. Let cool a bit in the baking dish before slicing into bars. Serve the bars while still warm, with the ice cream on top.

BLUEBERRY *crumble* BARS

TOTAL TIME: 1 HOUR **ACTIVE TIME:** 20 MINUTES **MAKES:** 10–12 BARS

For a short time after college I lived in Portland, Oregon. (I may or may not have moved there because of the abundance of vegan restaurants and farmer's markets.) One of my favorite things about living there (other than simply eating) was going to pick-your-own-berries farms on Sauvie Island. I still dream about those gorgeous berries. If there's anything better than freshly picked blueberries, it's this blueberry dessert.

DRY CRUMBLE
2 cups spelt flour
1 cup rolled oats
½ cup coconut sugar
½ teaspoon baking powder
½ teaspoon ground cinnamon
⅛ teaspoon salt

WET CRUMBLE
½ cup vegan butter or
    coconut oil, softened
¼ cup nondairy milk
2 teaspoons vanilla extract

BLUEBERRY FILLING
2 cups blueberries (fresh or
    frozen)
¼ cup coconut sugar
2 tablespoons cornstarch
Juice of 1 lemon

1. Preheat the oven to 350°F. Grease an 8-by-8-inch glass baking dish.

2. To prepare the crumble, whisk the dry crumble ingredients together in a large bowl. In a small bowl, stir the wet crumble ingredients together. Add the contents of the small bowl to the large bowl, and stir until mixed.

3. In a separate bowl, stir the blueberry filling ingredients together.

4. Use your hands to press about three-quarters of the crumble mixture into the bottom of the baking dish. Pour the blueberry filling on top and spread out evenly. Use your hands to break up the remaining crumble mixture and sprinkle it over the blueberry layer.

5. Bake for 45 minutes, until the top is crisp and bubbly. Let cool completely before slicing into bars, then serve or store in an airtight container.

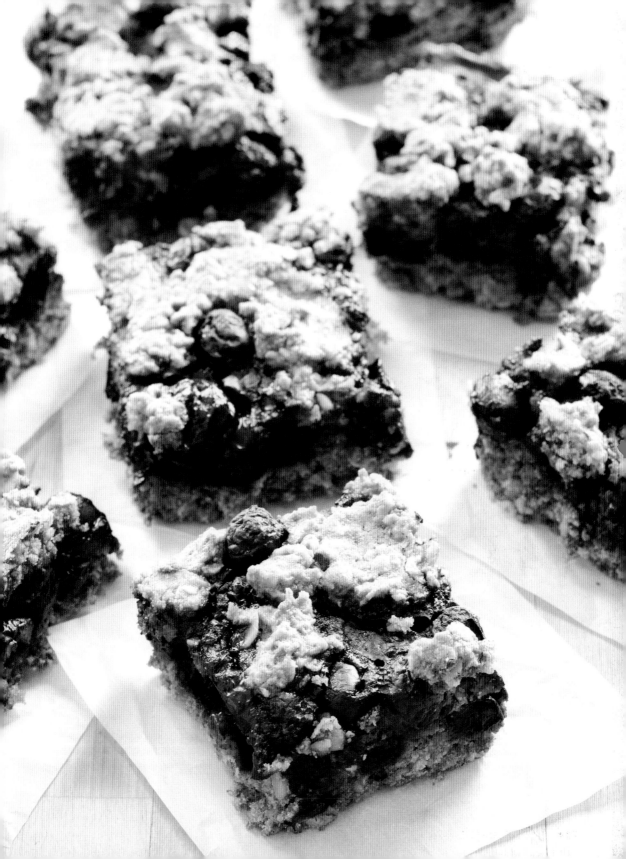

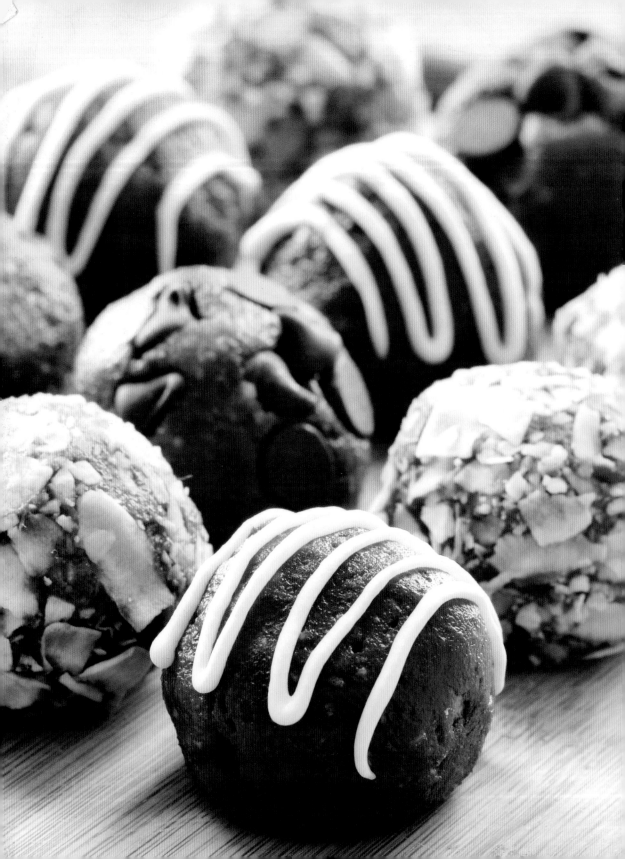

NO-BAKE CHIA *truffles*

TOTAL TIME: 20 MINUTES (PLUS TIME FOR SOAKING CASHEWS AND CHILLING)
MAKES: ABOUT 20 TRUFFLES

Dessert, power snack, or speedy breakfast—these sugar-free sweet treats are perfect for any time of the day.

TRUFFLES
1½ cups raw cashews, soaked in water at least 4 hours
1 cup Medjool dates, pitted and soaked in water 30 minutes
2 tablespoons chia seeds
2 tablespoons cocoa or cacao powder
2 tablespoons coconut oil, melted
Dash of salt

TOPPING OPTIONS
Shredded coconut
Cacao nibs
Chocolate chips
Coconut butter

1. Combine all the truffle ingredients together in a blender or food processor and blend until a mostly smooth texture is formed.

2. Line a baking sheet with wax paper. Using your hands, roll 1 tablespoon of batter into a ball, then place it on the baking sheet. Repeat until all the mixture is used.

3. Spread out your choice of toppings on individual plates. Roll the truffles around on the plates until they're coated, and use your hands to pat everything together. Use a spoon (or a pastry bag or a plastic baggie with a corner cut off) to drizzle the coconut butter over the truffles.

4. Place the truffles back on the baking sheet, and place in the refrigerator for about 1 hour to firm up before enjoying. Store in the refrigerator.

CHOCOLATE *banana* ICE CREAM SUNDAE

⊕ **TOTAL TIME:** 10 MINUTES **MAKES:** 4 SERVINGS

This recipe is similar to the Banana Breakfast Ice Cream Sundae (see page 21), but it's loaded up with a little extra indulgence. If you like soft serve, you need this totally decadent (and secretly wholesome) dessert in your life.

CHOCOLATE SAUCE
2 tablespoons maple syrup
2 tablespoons cocoa powder

ICE CREAM
4 frozen bananas*
¼ cup cocoa powder
Nondairy milk, as needed to blend
1–3 tablespoons maple syrup, to taste

TOPPINGS
1 batch Coconut Whipped Cream (see page 227)
¼ cup chopped walnuts
¼ cup cacao nibs
¼ cup shredded coconut

1. To prepare the chocolate sauce, stir the maple syrup and cocoa powder together in a small bowl. Set aside.

2. To prepare the ice cream, combine all the ingredients together in a blender or food processor and blend until smooth. Start with a couple of tablespoons of nondairy milk and add just enough to blend. The finished texture should be similar to that of frozen yogurt.

3. Transfer the ice cream to bowls. Top with the chocolate sauce and all the toppings. Enjoy right away.

NOTE: *See how to freeze bananas in the* **Colorful Ingredient Guide** *(page 16).*

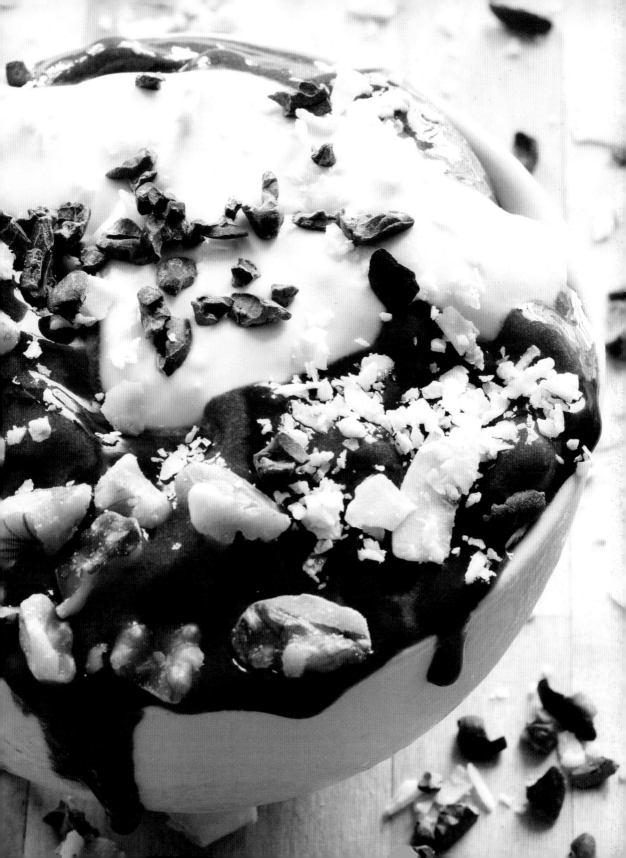

kitchen staples & sauces

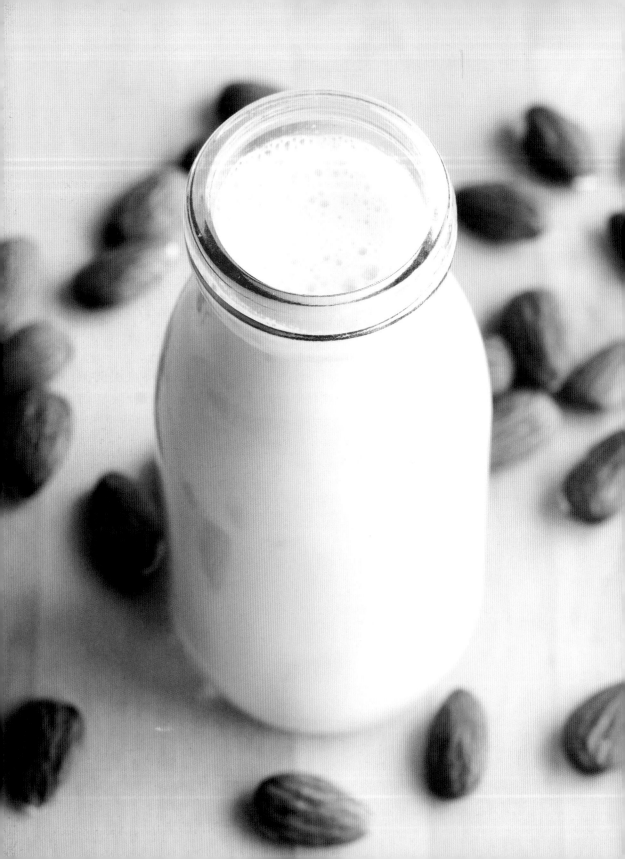

homemade
ALMOND MILK

TOTAL TIME: 10 MINUTES (PLUS TIME FOR SOAKING ALMONDS) **MAKES:** 4 CUPS

Many of the recipes in this book call for nondairy milk. You can find tons of varieties at the store (including many nut-free milks for those with allergies), but my personal favorite is homemade almond milk.

1 cup raw almonds, soaked in
   water overnight
4 cups water
1–2 Medjool dates, pitted
   (omit for unsweetened milk)
Dash of salt

1. Drain and rinse the almonds. Transfer them to a blender with the water, dates, and salt, and blend on high for at least 1 minute.

2. Strain the milk by pouring it through a nut milk bag* over a large bowl. The bag will catch the pulp and you'll be left with a smooth and creamy milk.

3. Transfer the milk to an airtight container and store in the refrigerator for up to 4 days.

NOTE: *You can find nut milk bags at most health-food stores or online.*

homemade VEGAN MAYO

TOTAL TIME: 5 MINUTES **MAKES:** 2 CUPS

Calling all sandwich lovers! This slightly tangy, egg-free mayo will help you build the perfect sandwich.

1 (14-ounce) package silken tofu
2 tablespoons olive oil
2 tablespoons apple cider vinegar
Juice of ½ lemon
1 teaspoon maple syrup
½ teaspoon dry mustard
½ teaspoon salt

1. Combine all the ingredients in a blender. Blend together until smooth. Transfer the mayo to an airtight container and store in the refrigerator for up to 1 week.

use in BKT (PAGE 105), CHICKPEA "TUNA" SALAD SANDWICH (PAGE 109), HARVEST BUTTERNUT SQUASH & APPLE BURGER WITH SAGE AIOLI (PAGE 177)

SWEET cashew CREAM

TOTAL TIME: 5 MINUTES (PLUS TIME FOR SOAKING CASHEWS) **MAKES:** 1 CUP

Made from just a few simple ingredients, this cashew cream is the perfect topping for any dessert, smoothie, or scoop of granola.

1 cup raw cashews, soaked in water at least 4 hours
2 tablespoons maple syrup
½ teaspoon vanilla extract
1–3 tablespoons nondairy milk

1. Drain and rinse the cashews. Transfer the cashews to a blender and add the maple syrup and vanilla extract.

2. Starting with 1 tablespoon at a time, add the nondairy milk as needed to blend, and blend until completely smooth. Transfer to an airtight container and store in the refrigerator for up to 5 days.

use in FRUITY BAKED OATMEAL (PAGE 39), PB&J SWEET CREAM TOAST (PAGE 42)

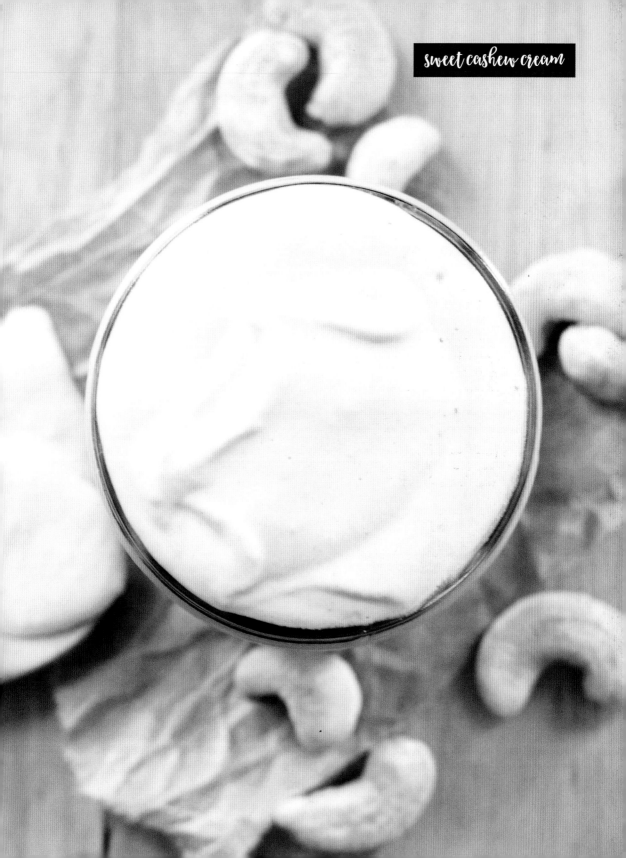

cashew SOUR CREAM

TOTAL TIME: 5 MINUTES (PLUS TIME FOR SOAKING CASHEWS) **MAKES:** 1 CUP

This savory cashew cream is great on just about every entrée in this book.

1 cup raw cashews, soaked in water at least 4 hours
Juice of ½–1 lemon, to taste*
2 teaspoons apple cider vinegar
1 teaspoon maple syrup
1–3 tablespoons nondairy milk
Salt and black pepper, to taste

1. Drain and rinse the cashews. Transfer the cashews to a blender and add the lemon juice, apple cider vinegar, and maple syrup.

2. Starting with 1 tablespoon at a time, add the nondairy milk as needed to blend, and blend until completely smooth. Add the salt and pepper and stir. Transfer to an airtight container and store in the refrigerator for up to 5 days.

NOTE: *Use a whole lemon for a tangier sour cream and a half lemon for a more mellow version.*

use in SOUTHWESTERN TOFU SCRAMBLE (PAGE 56), SWEET POTATO CHILI (PAGE 94), COCONUT-CRUSTED AVOCADO FRIES (PAGE 130), BALSAMIC BEET SPREAD (PAGE 143), SWEET POTATO SKINS (PAGE 173), CHEESY BROCCOLI & BACON STUFFED POTATOES (PAGE 174), PORTOBELLO & POTATO PESTO TACOS (PAGE 183)

COCONUT *whipped* CREAM

TOTAL TIME: 10 MINUTES (PLUS TIME FOR CHILLING COCONUT MILK)   **MAKES:** 1 CUP

When chilled in the refrigerator, the liquid and solid in cans of full-fat coconut milk will separate, giving us the gift of coconut cream. Just steer clear of reduced-fat versions and make sure not to skimp on refrigeration time.

1 (13½-ounce) can full-fat coconut milk, chilled in refrigerator at least 8 hours

1 tablespoon maple syrup

1. Open the can of coconut milk, drain the liquid on top, and scoop the cream out into a bowl.

2. Add the maple syrup and use a handheld or stand electric mixer to blend until a totally smooth, fluffy whipped-cream texture is formed. Enjoy fresh or store in an airtight container in the refrigerator for up to 5 days.

use in CHOCOLATE SUPERFOOD SMOOTHIE (PAGE 26), FRUITY BAKED OATMEAL (PAGE 39), NO-BAKE STRAWBERRY CHEESECAKE (PAGE 206), CHOCOLATE BANANA ICE CREAM SUNDAE (PAGE 218)

brown RICE

TOTAL TIME: 45 MINUTES **ACTIVE TIME:** 5 MINUTES **MAKES:** 4 SERVINGS

2¼ cups water or vegetable broth
1 cup brown rice
Dash of salt

1. In a medium pot, bring the water or vegetable broth to a boil over high heat. Add the rice and salt, reduce the heat to low, cover, and simmer for 40 minutes.

2. Turn the heat off and let the rice sit for 5 minutes before serving. If you are not using the rice right away, store it in an airtight container in the refrigerator for up to 4 days.

use in SPICY PEANUT & KIMCHI STEW (PAGE 101), VEGETABLE TERIYAKI STIR-FRY (PAGE 149), HARVEST BUTTERNUT SQUASH & APPLE BURGER WITH SAGE AIOLI (PAGE 177), BLACK BEAN BURGERS WITH TAHINI-MUSTARD SLAW (PAGE 179), REUBEN-ISH BOWL (PAGE 184), STEAMED GREENS & TOFU BOWL WITH MISO-GINGER SAUCE (PAGE 187)

quinoa

TOTAL TIME: 20 MINUTES **ACTIVE TIME:** 5 MINUTES **MAKES:** 4 SERVINGS

1 cup quinoa
2¼ cups water or vegetable broth
Dash of salt

1. Use a fine-mesh strainer to rinse the quinoa under running water (this removes the quinoa's coating, making it less bitter).

2. In a medium pot, bring the water or vegetable broth to a boil over high heat. Add the quinoa and salt, reduce the heat to low, cover, and simmer for 15 minutes.

3. Turn the heat off and let the quinoa sit for 5 minutes before serving. If you are not using the quinoa right away, store it in an airtight container in the refrigerator for up to 4 days.

use in SOUTHWESTERN SALAD WITH GREEN CASHEW RANCH DRESSING (PAGE 77), MUSHROOM QUINOA (PAGE 139), WHOLE ROASTED TAHINI CAULIFLOWER (PAGE 153)

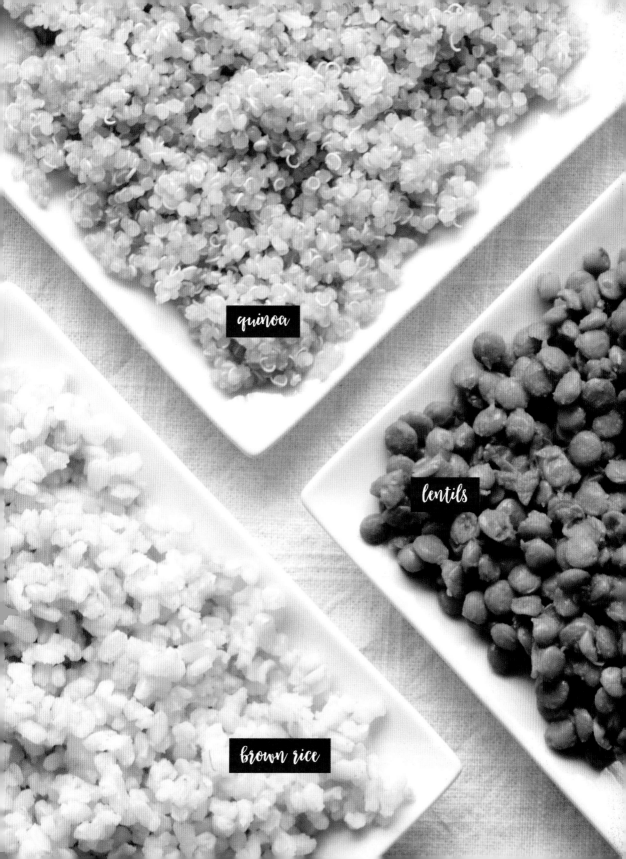

quinoa

lentils

brown rice

lentils

TOTAL TIME: 35 MINUTES   **ACTIVE TIME:** 5 MINUTES   **MAKES:** 4 SERVINGS

3 cups water or vegetable
   broth
1 cup lentils
Dash of salt

1. In a medium pot, bring the water or vegetable broth to a boil over high heat. Add the lentils and salt, reduce the heat to low, and simmer uncovered for about 30 minutes, until the water is absorbed. If you are not using the lentils right away, store them in an airtight container in the refrigerator for up to 4 days.

use in MEDITERRANEAN LENTIL SALAD WITH TOFU FETA (PAGE 82), SWEET POTATO SKINS (PAGE 173), MAPLE-MUSTARD SQUASH & LENTIL BOWL (PAGE 188)

tempeh BACON

TOTAL TIME: 30 MINUTES   **ACTIVE TIME:** 10 MINUTES   **MAKES:** 4 SERVINGS

This is my favorite easy way to prepare tempeh. It's perfect for tempeh beginners and you can add it to just about any meal.

MARINADE
1 tablespoon tamari
2 teaspoons olive oil
2 teaspoons liquid smoke
2 teaspoons vegan
   Worcestershire sauce
2 teaspoons maple syrup
½ teaspoon paprika
Dash of cayenne pepper
   (optional)

TEMPEH BASE
1 (8-ounce) package tempeh
1 tablespoon olive oil

1. Prepare the marinade by stirring all the ingredients together in a medium bowl.

2. Slice the tempeh lengthwise into strips about ⅓ inch thick, then cut the strips in half crosswise.

3. Add the tempeh to the bowl with the marinade and mix until the pieces are coated. Let the tempeh sit for at least 5 minutes—the longer, the better (overnight in the refrigerator is great).

4. Heat the olive oil in a pan over medium heat. Add the marinated tempeh and fry for about 5 minutes on each side, until browned. Enjoy right away or store in an airtight container in the refrigerator for up to 4 days.

use in ULTIMATE BREAKFAST SCRAMBLE SANDWICH (PAGE 59), BKT (PAGE 105), LOADED RANCH POTATO SALAD (PAGE 136), CHEESY BROCCOLI & BACON STUFFED POTATOES (PAGE 174)

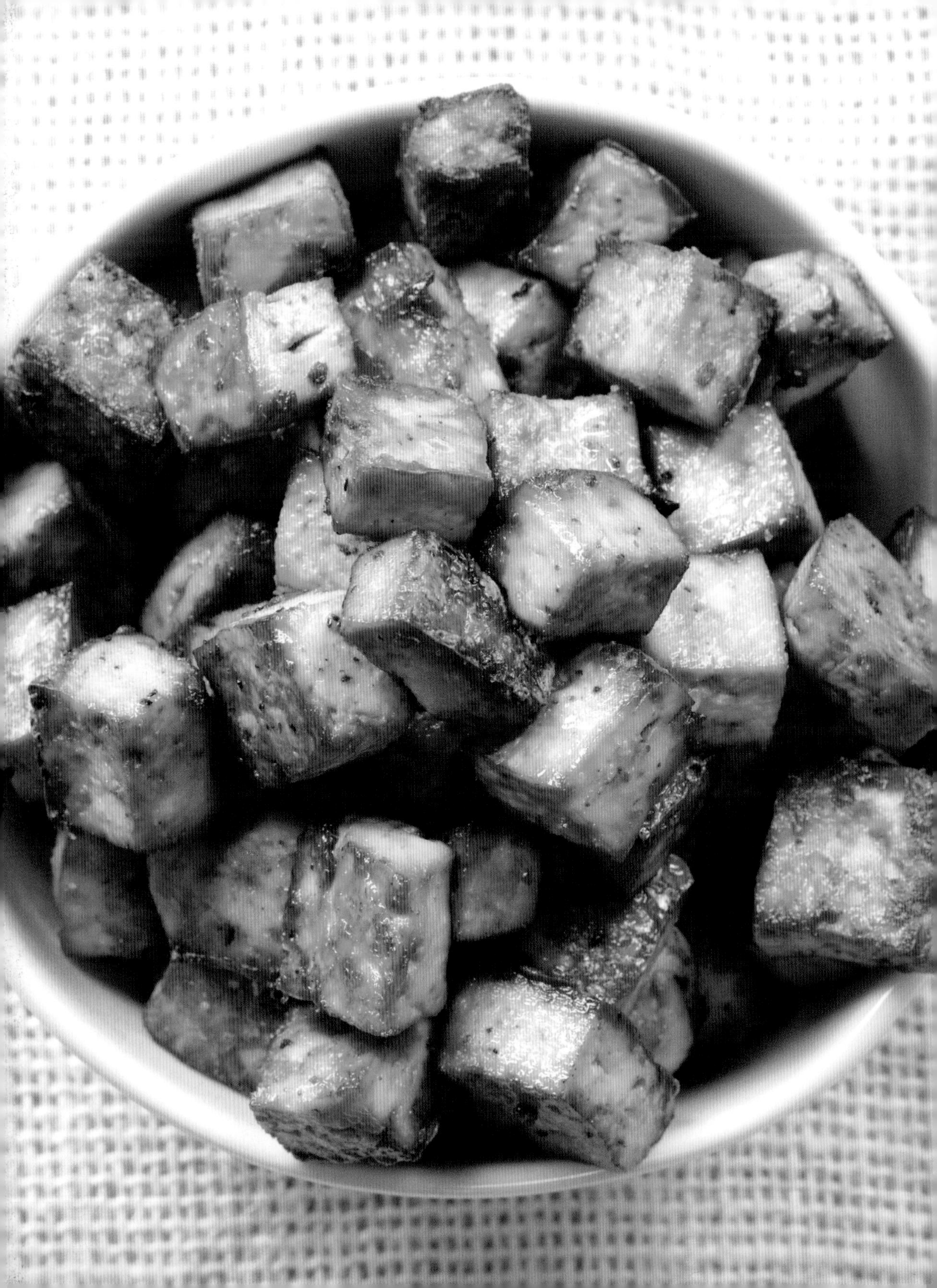

baked TOFU

TOTAL TIME: 1 HOUR (PLUS TIME FOR PRESSING TOFU) **ACTIVE TIME:** 10 MINUTES
MAKES: 4 SERVINGS

The key to preparing restaurant-quality tofu dishes at home is pressing the water out first. Thirty minutes will do the trick, but if you're able to plan ahead, a few hours (or even overnight in the fridge) will give your tofu a fantastic texture. Alternatively, for the recipes that call for Baked Tofu, you can buy pre-marinated and prebaked tofu. On especially busy weeks I'll go this route so I have a ready-to-go protein option.

1 (14-ounce) package firm tofu
1 tablespoon olive oil
1 tablespoon tamari
1 teaspoon rice vinegar
⅛ teaspoon garlic powder
⅛ teaspoon onion powder

1. Cut the tofu into ½- to 1-inch slices. On a cutting board, layer the slices of tofu between paper towels or clean dishcloths. Place a heavy item (a teakettle filled with water works great) on top (or use a tofu press if you've got one). Let the tofu sit for at least 30 minutes (or overnight in the refrigerator for extra-amazing texture). This will remove the excess water from the tofu and give it a better texture.

2. Preheat the oven to 400°F. Lightly grease a baking sheet.

3. To prepare the marinade, in a medium bowl, stir together the olive oil, tamari, rice vinegar, garlic powder, and onion powder. Leave the tofu as slices or cut it into cubes. Toss the tofu with the marinade in the bowl and let it soak for 5 minutes.

4. Spread the tofu out on the baking sheet. Bake for 15 minutes, then flip and bake for another 10–15 minutes (depending on the size of the pieces), until the desired crispiness is reached. Enjoy the tofu right away or store in an airtight container in the refrigerator for up to 4 days.

---

use in GRILLED REUBEN-ISH (PAGE 106), PINEAPPLE & PEANUT SAUCE TOFU WRAP (PAGE 110), VEGETABLE TERIYAKI STIR-FRY (PAGE 149), REUBEN-ISH BOWL (PAGE 184), STEAMED GREENS & TOFU BOWL WITH MISO-GINGER SAUCE (PAGE 187)

GREEN CASHEW *ranch* DRESSING

TOTAL TIME: 5 MINUTES (PLUS TIME FOR SOAKING CASHEWS)   **MAKES:** 1 CUP

1 cup raw cashews, soaked in water at least 4 hours
½ cup nondairy milk
Juice of 1 lemon
2 tablespoons chopped fresh parsley
2 tablespoons chopped fresh dill
1 tablespoon apple cider vinegar
1 teaspoon maple syrup
1 teaspoon garlic powder
1 teaspoon onion powder
Salt and black pepper, to taste

1. Drain and rinse the cashews. Transfer the cashews to a blender. Add the nondairy milk, lemon juice, parsley, dill, vinegar, maple syrup, garlic powder, onion powder, salt, and pepper. Blend until smooth. Store in an airtight container in the refrigerator for up to 5 days.

use in SOUTHWESTERN SALAD WITH GREEN CASHEW RANCH DRESSING (PAGE 77), BBQ CAULIFLOWER POPPERS (PAGE 135), LOADED RANCH POTATO SALAD (PAGE 136), BBQ RANCH CAULIFLOWER PIZZA (PAGE 170)

caesar DRESSING

TOTAL TIME: 5 MINUTES (PLUS TIME FOR SOAKING CASHEWS) **MAKES:** 1 CUP

1 cup raw cashews, soaked in water at least 4 hours
¼ cup nondairy milk
Juice of 1 lemon
2 tablespoons olive oil
1 tablespoon tamari
2 teaspoons Dijon mustard
1 teaspoon vegan Worcestershire sauce
1 clove garlic, crushed

1. Drain and rinse the cashews. Transfer the cashews to a blender. Add the nondairy milk, lemon juice, olive oil, tamari, mustard, Worcestershire sauce, and garlic. Blend until smooth. Store in an airtight container in the refrigerator for up to 5 days.

use in CRISPY CHICKPEA & KALE CAESAR SALAD (PAGE 75)

THOUSAND *island* DRESSING

TOTAL TIME: 5 MINUTES **MAKES:** 1 CUP

¼ cup vegan mayo, store-bought or homemade (see page 224)
1 tablespoon ketchup
1 teaspoon pickle brine
1 teaspoon maple syrup
⅛ teaspoon garlic powder

1. Stir all the ingredients together in a small bowl until smooth. Store in an airtight container in the refrigerator for up to 1 week.

use in GRILLED REUBEN-ISH (PAGE 106), REUBEN-ISH BOWL (PAGE 184)

peanut SAUCE

TOTAL TIME: 5 MINUTES **MAKES:** ½ CUP

¼ cup creamy peanut butter
2 tablespoons tamari
1 tablespoon rice vinegar
1 tablespoon sesame oil
1–2 tablespoons maple syrup,
   to taste
½ teaspoon garlic powder
Water, as needed to thin

1. Stir all the ingredients together in a small bowl until smooth. Store in an airtight container in the refrigerator for up to 1 week.

use in EDAMAME PEANUT NOODLE SALAD (PAGE 81), PINEAPPLE & PEANUT SAUCE TOFU WRAP (PAGE 110), AS SUBSTITUTE SAUCE IN VEGETABLE TERIYAKI STIR-FRY (PAGE 149)

KALE & *avocado* PESTO

TOTAL TIME: 5 MINUTES **MAKES:** 1 CUP

2 cups packed fresh basil
1 cup chopped kale
1 avocado, pitted and scooped
¼ cup olive oil
¼ cup chopped walnuts
1 tablespoon lemon juice
2 tablespoons nutritional yeast
2 cloves garlic, crushed
Salt and black pepper, to taste

1. Combine all the ingredients in a blender or food processor and pulse until a somewhat smooth but still slightly grainy texture is formed. Transfer to an airtight container and store in the refrigerator until ready to use. This pesto is best enjoyed fresh, so use within 2 days.

use in KALE & AVOCADO PESTO PASTA SALAD (PAGE 85), PORTOBELLO & POTATO PESTO TACOS (PAGE 183)

TERIYAKI *sauce*

TOTAL TIME: 5 MINUTES   **MAKES:** ½ CUP

¼ cup tamari
2 tablespoons brown rice syrup
2 teaspoons rice vinegar
1 teaspoon grated ginger
1 clove garlic, minced
2 teaspoons cornstarch

1. Whisk all the ingredients together in a small bowl until smooth. Store in an airtight container in the refrigerator for up to 1 week.

use in VEGETABLE TERIYAKI STIR-FRY (PAGE 149)

maple-mustard SAUCE

TOTAL TIME: 5 MINUTES   **MAKES:** ½ CUP

3 tablespoons olive oil
3 tablespoons maple syrup
2 tablespoons Dijon mustard
2 teaspoons tamari

1. Whisk all the ingredients together in a small bowl until smooth. Store in an airtight container in the refrigerator for up to 1 week.

use in MAPLE-MUSTARD SQUASH GRILLED CHEESE (PAGE 113), MAPLE-MUSTARD SQUASH & LENTIL BOWL (PAGE 188)

GREEN *tahini* SAUCE

TOTAL TIME: 5 MINUTES **MAKES:** ¾ CUP

½ cup tahini
Juice of 1 lemon
⅓ cup packed fresh parsley
3 tablespoons water
2 tablespoons olive oil
1 tablespoon tamari

1. Combine all the ingredients together in a blender or food processor and blend until smooth. Store in an airtight container in the refrigerator for up to 5 days.

use in HUMMUS BOWL WITH GREEN TAHINI SAUCE (PAGE 86), AS SUBSTITUTE SAUCE IN VEGETABLE TERIYAKI STIR-FRY (PAGE 149)

miso-ginger SAUCE

TOTAL TIME: 5 MINUTES **MAKES:** ¾ CUP

¼ cup sesame oil
2 tablespoons miso paste
1-inch piece ginger, grated
2 tablespoons tamari
2 tablespoons rice vinegar
2 tablespoons maple syrup

1. Whisk all the ingredients together in a small bowl until smooth. Store in an airtight container in the refrigerator for up to 1 week.

use in STEAMED GREENS & TOFU BOWL WITH MISO-GINGER SAUCE (PAGE 187)

CASHEW *cheese* SAUCE

TOTAL TIME: 5 MINUTES (PLUS TIME FOR SOAKING CASHEWS) **MAKES:** 1 CUP

1 cup raw cashews, soaked in water at least 4 hours
¼ cup plus 2 tablespoons nutritional yeast
Juice of ½ lemon
1 tablespoon Dijon mustard
1 tablespoon olive oil
1 tablespoon tamari
1 clove garlic, crushed
½ teaspoon ground turmeric (for color)
Nondairy milk, as needed to thin

1. Drain and rinse the cashews. Transfer the cashews to a blender. Add the nutritional yeast, lemon juice, mustard, olive oil, tamari, garlic, turmeric, and nondairy milk. Blend until smooth. Store in an airtight container in the refrigerator for up to 5 days.

use in AS SUBSTITUTE SAUCE IN VEGETABLE TERIYAKI STIR-FRY (PAGE 149), CHEESY BROCCOLI & BACON STUFFED POTATOES (PAGE 174), EGGPLANT & ZUCCHINI NO-NOODLE LASAGNA (PAGE 154)

CAULIFLOWER *alfredo* SAUCE

TOTAL TIME: 20 MINUTES **ACTIVE TIME:** 5 MINUTES **MAKES:** 2 CUPS

1 small cauliflower crown, broken into florets
1 cup nondairy milk
¼ cup nutritional yeast
2 tablespoons tamari
3 cloves garlic, crushed
Juice of 1 lemon
Salt and black pepper, to taste

1. Bring a large pot of water to a boil over high heat. Add the cauliflower and simmer until tender, 7–10 minutes. Drain the cauliflower and transfer it to a blender. Add the nondairy milk, nutritional yeast, tamari, garlic, lemon juice, salt, and pepper. Blend until smooth. Enjoy straight away or store in the refrigerator in an airtight container for up to 5 days.

use in AS SUBSTITUTE SAUCE IN VEGETABLE TERIYAKI STIR-FRY (PAGE 149), RAINBOW CAULIFLOWER ALFREDO PASTA (PAGE 165), CHICKPEA CRUST RAINBOW ALFREDO PIZZA (PAGE 166)

acknowledgments

To *The Colorful Kitchen* readers: without you this book would still be just a dream. I am endlessly grateful to each and every one of you for opening your computers and kitchens to me and my recipes.

To my literary agent, Christina Daignealt: you understood my vision for this book from the very start and I knew right away that I had to have you on my team. Thank you for guiding me through this process and being an unwavering source of support and confidence.

To my publisher, Glenn Yeffeth: I'm beyond grateful for the opportunity to write this book. Thank you to everyone at BenBella—Leah Wilson, Adrienne Lang, Heather Butterfield, Sarah Avinger, Alicia Kania, Jessika Rieck, Lindsay Marshall—for your guidance, creativity, and imagination.

To my editor, Maria Hart: thank you for working your magic over my manuscript, giving it unbelievably thorough care. You understood what I was trying to say when I couldn't find the words and were able to turn my nonsense into narrative.

Thank you to Jennifer Brett Greenstein for your incredibly thorough copyediting and to Kit Sweeney for the book's beautifully colorful interior design.

To my recipe testers, Julie Bedford, Danielle Drayer, Lindsay Elliott, Linda Geiler, April Hamlin, Caitlin Mack, Taryn Meyer, Alexi Sherrill, Megan Sutton, Jessica Turner, Katherine Wright, and Lynne Wright: thank you for the countless hours you spent testing the recipes in this book. They definitely did not all start out as winners, and your feedback was absolutely invaluable.

To my parents, Lynne and Eliot: thank you for always encouraging me to dream, and for supporting me through years and years of figuring it all out. I wouldn't be who I am today without our family dinners.

To my baby girl, Violet: thank you for being my sous-chef for nine months, even if being pregnant while writing this book almost made each recipe call for a side of pickles. All the hard work is worth it because of you.

To my husband, Ross: thank you for your endless love and support. You might not be the most discerning recipe tester, but you're the very best at doing the dishes.

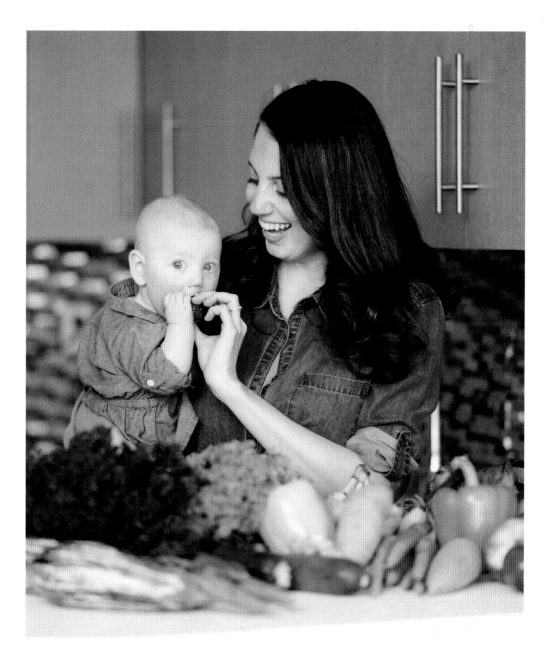

index

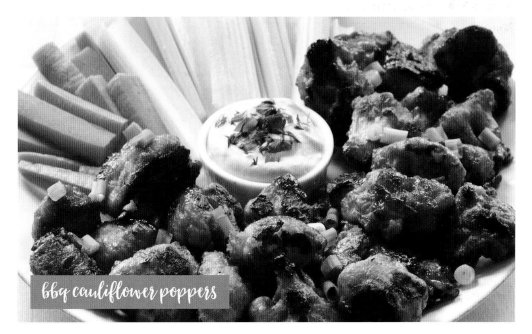

bbq cauliflower poppers

miso-tahini cookies

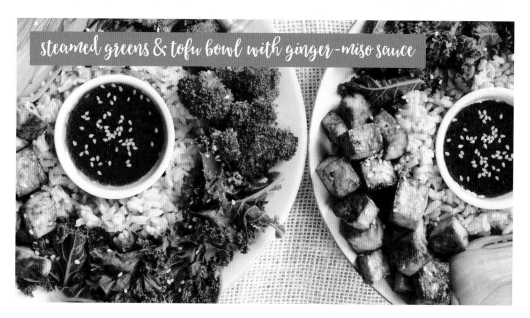

steamed greens & tofu bowl with ginger-miso sauce

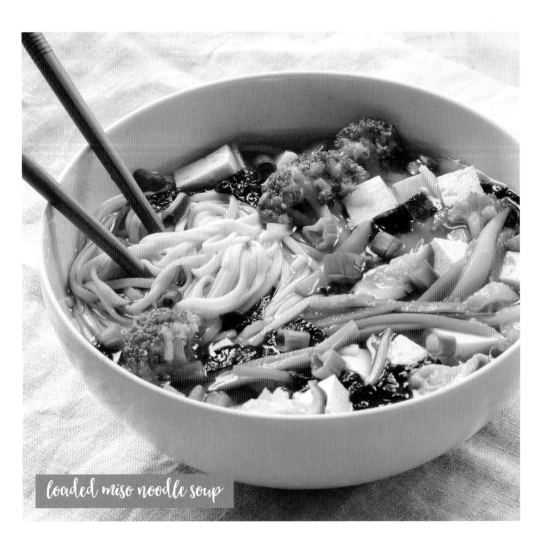

loaded miso noodle soup

pb&j sweet cream toast

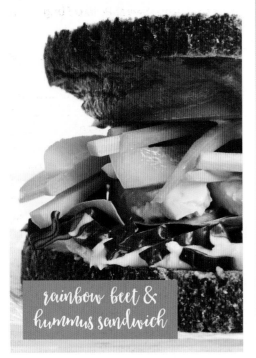

rainbow beet & hummus sandwich

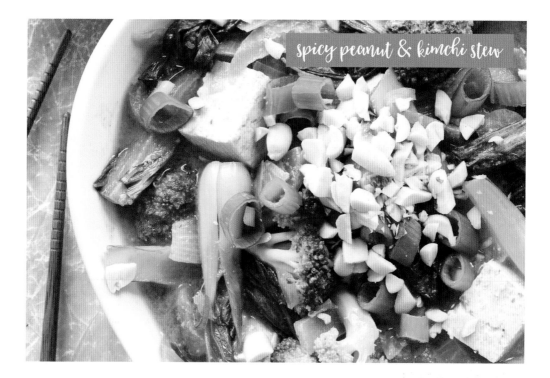

spicy peanut & kimchi stew

no-bake trail mix bars

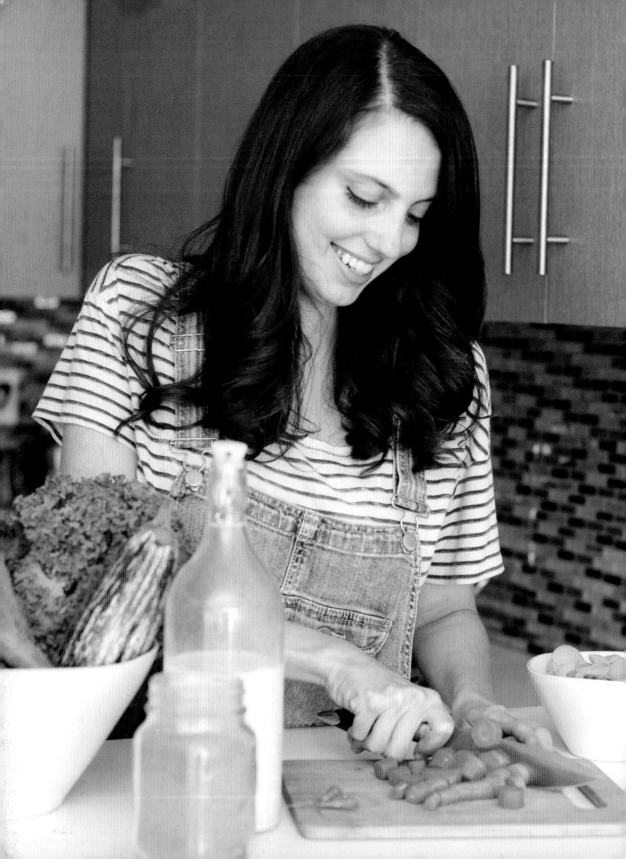

about
the author

Ilene Godofsky Moreno is a health coach, recipe developer, food photographer, and the gal behind the blog *The Colorful Kitchen*. She combines her background in design with her passion for plant-based food to create and share recipes that are "colorful, not complicated." Her recipes have been featured in the *New York Times*, *Huffington Post*, BuzzFeed, and *TODAY Food*, among others. Ilene can be found cooking and eating with her husband and daughter in her small (but colorful!) kitchen in Brooklyn, New York.

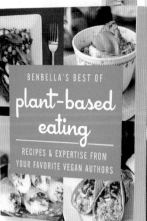
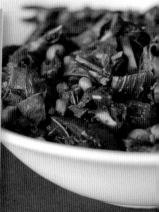